The Kitchen Witch Companion

Recipes, Rituals & Reflections

SARAH ROBINSON

LUCY H. PEARCE

Womancraft Publishing

Published by Womancraft Publishing, 2023
www.womancraftpublishing.com

ISBN 978-1-910559-90-1
The Kitchen Witch Companion is also available in ebook format: ISBN 978-1-910559-89-5

Cover design, interior design and typesetting: lucentword.com

Cover image © Jessica Roux, jessica-roux.com
Illustrations: Lucy H. Pearce

Womancraft Publishing is committed to sharing powerful new women's voices, through a collaborative publishing process. We are proud to midwife this work, however the story, the experiences and the words are the author's alone. A percentage of Womancraft Publishing profits are invested back into the environment reforesting the tropics (via TreeSisters) and forward into the community.

Medical disclaimer

We mention within these pages all sorts of thrilling herbs and flowers from ancient texts and old folklore. But please, for the love of goddess, use care if you go out foraging for houndstongue, pinks and nettles. When it comes to gathering herbs and foods from the wild you need to be very careful and know exactly the plant you are seeking, and what you intend to do with it. If in any doubt at all, seek a wise one, be they herbalist, witch, forager or chef.

Praise for *The Kitchen Witch Companion*

This is the sort of book you need to be reading in front of an open fire with a cup of coffee and a slice of cake. Taking your time so that you can truly appreciate the wonderful content. The authors have come together to create a beautiful book on the amazing art of Kitchen Witchcraft. Pull up a chair and put the kettle on, you are in for a real treat.

Rachel Patterson, English Kitchen Witch and High Priestess of the Kitchen Witch Coven, author of over twenty-five books on witchcraft including *Grimoire of a Kitchen Witch* and the *Kitchen Witchcraft* series

The true grail isn't found in castles guarded by knights, it was secretly hidden in the original place of magic, the womb of the home, the feminine alchemy lab, the center – the kitchen. Guarded by wise- women, soup-stirrers, and tea-scryers, practitioners of feminine magic hid their deepest secrets in pots and pans and kettles and coded their manuscripts in recipes. In this beautiful book, Lucy and Sarah invite you in for a cup of tea and bite to eat, to restore the power of the hearth and home where it belongs, not to fantasy housewives, but to rooted, generous women of magic and power, who know how to stir the pot in the right direction, how to feed the soul, nourish the body and celebrate everyday ceremony.

Seren Bertrand, author of *Spirit Weaver*, co-author of Womb Awakening and *Magdalene Mysteries*

Practical, healing and celebratory, this gorgeous collaboration is a wonderful weaving of kitchen- witch wordsmithery which will accompany you on an enchanting journey through the alchemical abundance of recipes and rituals.

Beautiful and brilliant.

It inspires.

It invokes.

It informs.

And it beckons you to the reality of everyday magic.

Veronika Sophia Robinson, author of the plant-based recipe books *The Mystic Cookfire* and *Love from My Kitchen*

This newest instalment of Kitchen Witch is such a bountiful gift. A book for life that will be much used in my home, taking pride of place on an easily accessible kitchen shelf. Stuffed full of wisdom and magical kitchen based power shared with warmth and ease. Like an inspired hug from all our ancestral Grandmothers which imparts a cauldron of helpful, deep practice and knowing.

Alice Grist, author of *Soulful Pregnancy* and *Dirty & Divine*

OTHER BOOKS BY THE AUTHORS

Sarah Robinson

Yoga for Witches
Yin Magic: How to be Still
Kitchen Witch: Food, Folklore & Fairy Tale
Enchanted Journeys: Guided Meditations for Magical Transformation

Lucy H. Pearce

The Rainbow Way
Moon Time: living in flow with your cycle
Reaching for the Moon: a girl's guide to her cycles
Moods of Motherhood: the inner journey of mothering
Full Circle Health: integrated health charting for women
Burning Woman
Medicine Woman: reclaiming the soul of healing
Creatrix: she who makes
She of the Sea
Crow Moon: reclaiming the wisdom of the dark woods

CONTENTS

INTRODUCTION

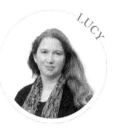

The drive to create *The Kitchen Witch Companion* came about when I was editing Sarah's third book, *Kitchen Witch*. The idea for it has been brewing since I worked on her very first book, *Yoga for Witches*. There was a whole section of recipes in the first draft that were gorgeous... but didn't quite fit, as well as a chapter called Kitchen Witch! "That needs to be a book in its own right," I told her. And so it is – as a joint effort – nearly five years later!

I have loved working with Sarah on her books as her editor and publisher over the past few years. Books which have turned out to be the biggest sellers in Womancraft's herstory. So what a treat to work on one shoulder-to-shoulder together as authors.

Some readers may know me as the author of many books. As Sarah's editor, however, my work goes unseen, but what we do together behind the scenes to bring a manuscript from draft to finished book is a little like cooking together... we chop and stir, season and taste, and finally serve together.

Sarah is loved for her witch books and magical writing. Me for archetypes and creativity. Both of us have a passion for the seasons, foraging and food.

Not many people know that my first writing dream was actually to be a cookery writer. Age seven I used to present my own cookery radio shows in the playground. At nine I wrote my first cookery book as a gift for my stepmother. At eighteen I wrote to my favourite cookery authors asking how to get started in cookery book writing. I was so grateful to get a handwritten reply from the domestic goddess, Nigella, herself! At twenty when studying History of Ideas and English Literature I, of course, chose to study the course on food in literature.

However, I soon realised that whilst I love cooking and sharing food, and I love writing, our local area did not need another cookery writer (I live in a village of around a thousand inhabitants of which six are cookery book authors!) The world does not need another version of cottage pie in a glossy magazine. I had the privilege of working alongside esteemed Irish cookery author Darina Allen, proofreading the recipes for one of her books, and for many years working on her blog as well as copywriting for her cookery school website. I was the cookery contributor at Juno magazine for about eighteen months. I love writing about what food means to us... "food as a connective force, a source of strength and joy" (Nina Mingya Powles, *Small Bodies of Water*). My favourite writing about food happened on two of my blogs – Dreaming Aloud and The Queen of Puddings – and in published pieces in *The Guardian* and the BlogHer food anthology at the very beginning of my writing career.

I love the magic of food, the alchemy of ingredients, occasion, season and people... and evoking that with words. I love incorporating meaning and symbolism into my food. I use food and cooking to help me feel calm, to feel safe, to celebrate and nourish those I love. I am a feeder. I love the way food and cooking help me feel connected to places I have been, people I love who are far away or no longer here: the way that cooking their food conjures them up through flavour and memory. Food – gathering, making eating and writing about it – holds great magic for me.

When my creative and spiritual energy is engaged in making art or writing, my cooking is naturally more perfunctory. Much of the time kitchen magic is getting food on the table ten minutes after we get in the door from a busy day. Sometimes it's feeding lots of mouths from almost nothing, making a little go a long way. Whereas on weekends, at key seasonal times, when I am between projects, I pour my energy into more conscious magic making, spell craft, creating sustenance, healing and celebrating the seasons in my kitchen, through food.

This project has been a way for me to celebrate kitchen magic in so many ways: through conjuring words, creating images of beloved plants, thinking and reading about food magic, connecting with other women who feel the same, asking them to share their skills and secrets… and most of all cooking: remembering old recipes, trying new foraged wonders like magnolia, honeysuckle and flowering currant.

Over time, the food side of my work has fallen by the wayside in my writing, though you will occasionally see my kitchen magic appear on my Instagram feed. It has been such a delight to work on this book with Sarah, to write consciously and explicitly about the aspects of food that excite me most, the unseen energetics that I have previously only reflected on privately. A tsunami of words and images has emerged from me. I did not know that I was this hungry to write this book. To do so with Sarah has been a joy, an honour and a privilege. We have complimentary skills and the power of a thousand books pumping through our veins. I hope *The Kitchen Witch Companion* brings you as much joy as it has us.

Lucy is an inspiration, to me, and to pretty much anyone who's ever read her books or heard her speak. I had her books on my shelves for years before I one day submitted my own book proposal to Womancraft Publishing. And it was Lucy who saw the potential of more detail on kitchen witchery drawn from just few lines in my first book, and then from the full-blown book that those lines became in *Kitchen Witch* – still, there is more possibility, more magic to be found! Lucy is skilled in seeing potential where I cannot, and I am eternally grateful for that!

I am honoured to have the very best of help. I was thrilled to learn that Lucy has a passion and long legacy of writing recipes and editing cookbooks, which means at least one of us knows what we're up to!

Neil Gaiman once said that Terry Pratchett inviting him to work on a book together was like Michelangelo saying, "Hey, want to do a ceiling with me?" I feel the same, of course I wasn't going to turn down this chance to work with Lucy when she proposed it! But it has presented me with challenges (all my own creation, of course!) I don't always like being in the kitchen and I've never successfully followed a recipe in my life! I felt unworthy to the challenge of co-authoring.

I have said to Lucy several times during the creation of this book "but I'm shit at recipes!" even though, as she so sagely pointed out, I have managed to work recipes into every one of the Womancraft books I have written, and even several ebook projects too. Somewhere the love and fantasy of the magic in the kitchen doesn't always connect with my day-to-day workings in the kitchen where I am largely grumpy, harried and rushed, lamenting almost every day that this is an hour I could be writing in, instead I'm cooking dinner!

But I suppose that is the point of these kitchen stories – they are imperfect. We are, so often within the kitchen, stressed, hot, frustrated, some things don't work out how we hoped they would. Sometimes (like many other people, I am sure) I hate cooking and hate my messy kitchen. And it's curses, not charms, I throw about as I clatter pots and pans. But then my beloved will give me a hug, and we'll pour a glass of wine, and get dinner from the chippy. Or I remind myself how lucky I am to have someone to cook for. Or maybe we carry some cold beers round to our friends who have two children under two… and let them enjoy a drink and adult conversation! In a way it couldn't be farther from the witches and their bubbling cauldrons of healing herbs. In a way it's just the same – coming together for connection, comfort, a few laughs, and it doesn't really matter if that involves burnt sausages and failed desserts. Fortified with favourite foods and drinks, we are revived and able to start again.

This book is an opportunity for me and Lucy to weave together some of our passions with the beautiful words of others. So, as Lucy says, we are cooking together, bringing in recipes of our own and of others. She is drawing on vast experience and knowledge, and I'm so busy talking that I've put in the wrong spices and dropped a spoon with a splash of sauce all over the floor… But when the time comes, like all good party hostesses, we've got libations in hand, music is playing gently in the background, the candles are lit. Welcome, dear ones! Come in, grab a glass of whatever you want and a slice of cake, and join us, we are thrilled have so much joy, magic and glorious imperfection to share!

WHAT'S IN STORE?

Within this book there are real people, real recipes, real practices grounded in lived experience and the very real lives of those who find comfort, connection and ancestral honouring within crafts and rituals based around the kitchen sphere. It shares the living breathing practice of just some of the diverse contemporary kitchen witches who are making everyday magic in their homes. We share reflections, recipes and rituals to help you deepen your practice of cooking as a magical art and help you to (re)discover what you are hungry for, in your life, and home, encouraging and empowering you to conjure that up for yourself.

Kitchen witchcraft is, in essence, the magic of hearth, home and food. And the term enjoys many positive associations. The kitchen is where we all once gathered, shared knowledge, discovered the secrets and alchemy of plants, created remedies, and became the first healers, nurses, midwives and early physicians. We learned how to nourish and sustain ourselves and our families, transferring skills and gaining knowledge. Modern cooking has become more about calories in or calories avoided, about politics, efficiency and showboating gadgets and techniques. We have to eat to live, but many of us have lost our why: food not only as nourishment, but as something that acts in spiritual and symbolic ways as well. In short, food as magic.

You don't need to publicly, or even privately, identify as a witch to enjoy this book. There is nothing you need to believe. You can celebrate sabbats or not, have a cat, cauldron and ceremonial broomstick… or not. There are no satanic practices here, no curses, hexes or black magic. We have sought to create an eclectic and accessible set of resources, with only a passing reference to Wicca and its specific rites and goddesses, glorious as they are for many. We seek to allow space for every recipe and every sacred practice in its own right, space for the trees to be our deities, the wildflowers our seasonal wheel and perhaps to find our own rhythm free from rules.

 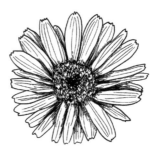

The Kitchen Witch Companion is about understanding the magic that lies beneath the acts of cooking, gathering and celebrating in your kitchen, so that you can deepen your enjoyment and engage more consciously with what you are doing, picking up nuggets of insight and new recipes or ideas to try. We hope that this will make your experience of cooking and celebrating the seasons richer, and that it encourages you to share this with others who enjoy it. We want to help you find and make meaningful celebrations of your own within your own community, rather going through the motions of prescribed cultural holidays focused on commercialism. Our intention is to bring you back to the heart of what and why we celebrate – alone and together – how we do it through food, rooting your rituals back to the heart of the home, the kitchen, and connected to your heart and imagination, to *your* ancestors and the land.

We start by reflecting on the roots and lived experience of what kitchen magic looks like, in fantasy and reality, the archetypes of the Kitchen Witch, Domestic Goddess and Housewife and a little of their history. We explore what magic is and how and why we might make it as well as the alchemy of cooking. Then, in the second part, we share our personal favourite seasonal recipes for celebrating with family and friends and treasured ways to preserve nature's abundant foraged bounty, as well as crafts and rituals to celebrate the seasons of

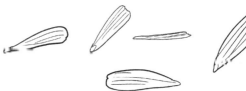

year and life from our contributing coven of kitchen witches. This is a compendium of delights, of everyday magic-making with recipes to heal and nourish body and soul.

If you read and loved Sarah's previous book, *Kitchen Witch: Food, Folklore & Fairy Tale,* we know you will be excited to hear that we include many of the traditional recipes referenced in there: bannocks, butter, colcannon, May wine, rose petal jam, mulled wine, gingerbread and mince pies. We hope this will be a book that you enjoy reading in the bedroom or on your sofa and cooking from in the kitchen, that will inspire you to go out into the garden, market, park, hedgerows, fields or forests to gather in the goodness.

This book shares practices, recipes and insights that have been guides, supports, treasures and portals for us in accessing magic, healing and delight in our own lives. Our dearest hope is that even one might offer a way back to remembering your magic… and bringing it into the world through the sanctuary space of your own kitchen.

MEET THE CONTRIBUTORS – OUR KITCHEN WITCH COVEN

This book is a collective endeavour, a sharing of diverse practices from diverse kitchen witches. We noticed that so many books about witchcraft and ritual are written by a single author, from a single perspective. Whilst each of us has insights we have learned from our own teachers – mothers, grandmothers, aunts, friends, mentors – the wisdom of kitchen witchery is communal and collectively held. This is how the practice of kitchen witchery has always happened: passed-on recipes written on the back of envelopes, copied from treasured recipe books, rituals practiced together and adapted. This is how our own practice has developed, and how we hope you will work with the material we share here. Make it your own. Get creative. Allow your magic to be personal, your ritual intuitive. There is nothing set in stone.

Just as we open a women's circle with a check in, so we shall here, so that you get to meet our virtual community, and see how we are scattered around the globe, each in our own kitchen, apart but together, brewing magic and gathering goodness. We each have our areas of experience and even expertise. We are all in this circle together, inspiring each other, cheering each other on, sharing hints and tips, passing round the cake, slipping a recipe into your bag as you leave.

The act of moving from writing separately to weaving our voices together on the page has been a wonderful creative venture. Most of the time the main authors Lucy and Sarah speak as one. But we both have personal stories, memories and experiences to share, and have done so by placing our pictures next to our stories.

The other voices from our coven are named after their contribution. In order to be true to each voice, we have maintained our American authors' US spelling throughout the book.

Alice Tarbuck is an academic, writer and literature professional based in Edinburgh, Scotland. She holds a BA and MPhil in English Literature from Emmanuel College, Cambridge, and a doctorate from the University of Dundee. She writes about her experiences as a modern witch and practices what she describes as 'intersectional, accessible' witchcraft. Her best-known work is *A Spell in the Wild: A Year (and six centuries) of Magic.* Website: alicetarbuck.net

Coco Oya Cienna-Rey is a UK-based creative, mystic and writer based in the UK. Her creativity is informed by her journey as a devotee of the Tantric path. She has always felt a call to channel the voice of the Divine Feminine and is published in several anthologies. Often thought-provoking, always heartfelt, her work speaks of the sacred wisdom stored in the body, the non-linear nature of trauma and the embodiment of soul. She can be found weaving her soul-coaching embodiment work out in the world at creativelycoco.com

Indra Roelants lives in Cork, Ireland, in Sunflower House, in the middle of an old garden centre. She is currently juggling working full time for a global corporation, whilst re-starting the garden centre and raising three children, three cats, a dog and twelve hens. The power of mother nature and all She provides is central to her everyday life and the kitchen is the very heart of Sunflower House.
   Website: stonewallgardencentre.com

Jacqueline Durban is a writer and poet living in a hedgehermitage by the sea on the South Coast of England. She believes in small beauties, wild hope, and the quiet magic of a nice cup of tea. She is hedgevicar of the Little Church of Love of the World, and can be found at linktr.ee/jacquelinedurban

Jessica M. Starr is a storyweaver, poet, and stargazer. She lives under the oak trees on the edge of a village, in her ancestral homeland of South Wales, with her musician husband, their two unschooled children, and Frodo the little white dog. Jessica is the author of *Waking Mama Luna* and *Maid Mother Crone Other.* When she's not foraging in the woods you can find her on her YouTube channel Jessica and the Moon. Website: jessicamstarr.com / Instagram: @thestorywitch

Khyati Patel is an aspiring clinical psychologist, she is interested in all things related to mental health. Her love for food comes from growing up eating delicious generational recipes cooked by her mum and maternal grandmother to help her feel more connected to her Indian roots whilst growing up in London. Khyati firmly believes that food is the magic that connects all around the table.

Leigh Millar is a mum of three living in a little cottage by the sea in the south of Ireland, and a much-loved and valued member of the Womancraft team. Leigh loves to support her and her family's health with herbs from her garden where she welcomes all 'weeds' and wildflowers. But most of all she loves to bake and share the results with her friends!

Milly Watson Brown is the creatress of Moon Time Chocolate, based in Devon, England. She hand-crafts delicious chocolate truffles with herbs, flowers and oils to support the menstrual cycle, new mums and the menopause. She makes a lot of her own tinctures for the chocolates, with wild crafted herbs. Website: moontimechocolate.co.uk / Instagram: @moontimechocolate

Molly Remer, MSW, D.Min, is a priestess, mystic, and poet in central Missouri. Molly and her husband Mark co-create Story Goddesses at Brigid's Grove. Molly is the author of ten books, including *Walking with Persephone, Whole and Holy, Womanrunes,* the *Goddess Devotional,* and *365 Days of Goddess.* She is the creator of the devotional experience #30DaysofGoddess and she loves savouring small magic and everyday enchantment.
   Website: Brigidsgrove.com / Instagram @brigidsgrove

Penny Allen lives in East Cork, Ireland with her husband and daughters surrounded by their two acres of rewilded garden. She set up the Fermenting Shed at Ballymaloe Cookery School in 2018 where they make water kefir, kombucha and sauerkraut, supplying the shop and cookery school. Penny enjoys introducing the students to the alchemy of fermentation and holds workshops throughout the year. She walks with her dog Oscar everyday communing with trees and plants along the way!
   Ballymaloe Cookery School website: cookingisfun.ie

Sarah Napoli, also known as The Woodland Witch, is a practicing folk witch, herbalist and witchy mom located in the heart of New England, USA. It has been her passion to share her herbal knowledge and magic with others, which led her to open her business Folkcraft and Flora Apothecary where she crafts potions, brews and herbal remedies to help others utilise the benefits of plants and craft a little bit of magic of their own.
   Website: folkcraftandflora.com / Instagram: @thewoodlandwitchh

And you are a treasured part of our circle now.
   We hope this collection of recipes, rituals and reflections brings you colour, beauty, inspiration and lots of magic.

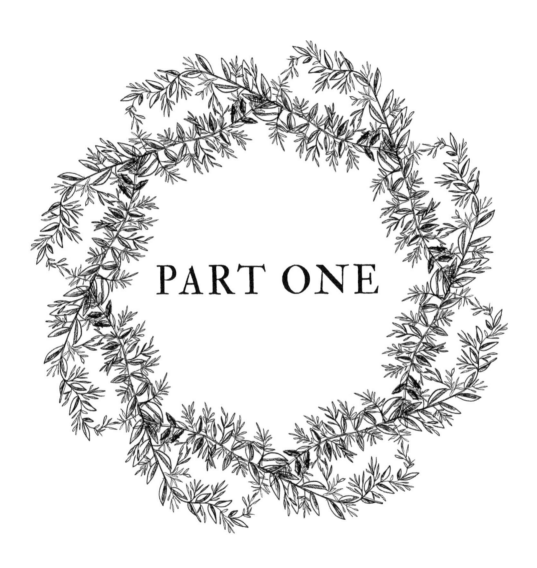

PART ONE

Stir in hope
Season with love
Eat with joy

HUNGRY FOR MAGIC

Once we wove magic… we held it in our hands, we created it from scraps, we saw it in signs and portents, we baked it into pies and held it in offerings for deities and our dear departed. We crafted charms for our hearths and the creation of food was held in reverence and honoured in rituals, for we were magical women and all the magic to see, feel, create was already within us. Then, slowly, insidiously, these ways were cast out, overlooked, punished by a patriarchal society that could not believe that women should own such power, know such things, be connected in such unknowable ways. So magic, for many, was distrusted, demonised and cast away. Those who worked with magic were forced to step away from it. And so here we are in the present day, where talking of magic is not so easy…

We live in a culture that claims not to believe in magic. And yet we are exhorted to expend vast amounts of energy and resources in trying to create it for culturally approved celebrations: Christmas, Valentine's Day, Easter, birthdays, weddings, christenings… The days of preparation required to cook, decorate for and host the major festivals, still falls largely to women. And it's not only the physical work that falls on our shoulders, but the spiritual and emotional aspects of care, love, and intuitive insight that when combined make an occasion magical and meaningful. This is work that is not valued, which must by necessity go unseen, so as not to break the illusion, as we conjure the magic of Santa, the Easter Bunny, the Tooth Fairy, and the Elf on the effing Shelf.

And oh, how we have seen that insidious devaluing of women's carework played out through the decades: the scientists in white coats visiting new mothers in hospital with their formula, claiming it to be far superior to the breast milk she created herself. Because how could a woman's body possibly create something better than modern science? The zero calorie drinks* and powdered soups advised as replacements for home-made breads and soups, because why be nourished and satiated when you can seek to be thinner? And the generations of women scoffed at, derided, insulted for hanging a charm in her kitchen or brewing elderberry tinctures every winter to ward off colds. (When she knows full well the origin of the aspirins you are popping instead.†) The shame instilled onto healers when an aggressive challenger demands to know: *where's the science behind this?* As if centuries of learned knowledge are a lesser form of proof.

We were born with hearts and minds open to the possibility of magic and wonder, then, at a certain age we are shamed for believing in magic. We grow into a place of paradox: the paradox that women must make magical experiences, but women who claim that power of making magic are silly, strange, even dangerous.

As good girls of the patriarchy, we have been taught to force ourselves into overdrive in order to deliver socially approved magic, elegance, ease and service for others – in our homes and workplaces – all the while overlooking our own needs, limitations or desires. As a society, we are buying more and

---

* These foods are not necessarily bad – an ice-cold fizzy drink can be a joy on a hot day – but they are certainly not nourishing.

† From the trees, like many of our oldest medicines.

more to cover the cracks made by a complete disconnection of what it actually means to hold food and family and nature as sacred things. A hundred brightly wrapped gifts seeking to evoke the joy that was once found in the rituals and songs sung for centuries, passed through families around the hopes and joys of rekindled fires.

We believe that many of us are tired of this consumption that does not truly feed us. We are seeing more clearly what we sacrifice in the name of that consumption. However well-fed we may be, we believe there is a part of every one of us that is hungry for more. Hungry for magic – to see it in the world around us, to feel its power in ourselves, to know it as real. We may have packed this part away with childhood dreams and deny it, we may nourish it with fiction and fantasy, or indulge it with luxurious fripperies that sparkle. But still it remains: a hunger to have faith once more in our own power of magic. Hunger to once more see cooking as one of the most valuable acts of care, and to honour the benefits of growing and gathering as a path to well-being and healing. But this is no call to be chained to the kitchen sink or in any way feel trapped in the kitchen – we may well also hunger to have our effort appreciated, seen, honoured. To choose to make our way into the kitchen or out into the wildwood to forage for supper. Or to revel in the magic of warm meals with friends. We hunger most of all to live with purpose and to own our choices, whatever they may be, to bring a powerful intentionality to our time in (or out of) the kitchen.

If women trusted and claimed their desires, the world as we know it would crumble.
Perhaps that is precisely what needs to happen so we can rebuild truer,
more beautiful lives, relationships, families, and nations in their place.
Maybe Eve was never meant to be our warning.
Maybe she was meant to be our model.
Own your wanting.
Eat the apple.

Glennon Doyle, *Untamed*

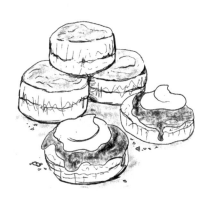

We are taught to ignore our appetites in many ways: through diet culture and body shaming. We are taught not to fantasise and dream for too much, for more, for a life beyond dross and drudgery. We are taught in a thousand different ways to settle for less, not to go for what we truly desire. Be that the creamy dessert on the menu or following our passions.

When did you learn to distrust your hunger? What do you do with it instead?

"A witch," author Ray Bradbury once wrote, "is born out of the true hungers of her time."*

This, for us, is a profoundly insightful observation. The idea of Witch feeds the needs of both a culture and an individual, often in paradoxical ways: as a representative of the mysterious and powerful feminine. Her power is both longed for and distrusted. Her wisdom needed and feared. Her magic denied and desired.

For centuries the reality and fantasy of the witch have blurred with the patriarchy's fear (and need and desire) of women. Women learned that to be perceived as powerful was too dangerous: to follow our inner guidance above external rules could mean death. If you are interested in exploring this history of women and witchcraft more this is a topic that both of us have written passionately about in our other books, Lucy in *Burning Woman*, and Sarah in *Kitchen Witch*.

We believe what we are hungry for in our time is meaning, purpose, connection and magic. We are bloated by domestication and longing for the wild. We have become disenchanted with the way things are: hungry for more.

In a world caught in 24-hour news cycles of death, destruction, ecological and political doom we can regularly feel powerless, hopeless and disconnected from each other, nature and ourselves. We long for the ability to heal those we love, and ourselves. We yearn to feel more fully alive. We are longing to remember, to recover something deep that has been lost. This, we believe, is what the resurgence of modern witchcraft represents: a reclaiming of other ways – old and new approaches to more meaningful, magical, wild and wonderful ways of being.

The inner witch – the wise woman within – is always trying to get back to the world beyond this world, the reality beyond this reality, to true meaning. She sniffs the air for its scent. She follows its ways in her dreams. She hungers for more. But still we smell the smoke of the women burned as witches and know we must be cautious. And so begins the inner battle between feeding the inner witch and starving her. Most inner witches are starving: a hungry witch is a dangerous creature!

And so we ask you: What do you hunger for, dear one? What are your body and soul yearning for? What is missing in your daily life? Connection, mindfulness, power, vitality, slowness, wildness, joy, wonder, a sense of enchantment or peace? Have you ever experienced these? If so, can you remember how or why they were lost? Are you able to awaken and heed the rich creative resources of your imagination and fantasy? Are you ready to feed yourself what you are longing for?

Here at the crossroads of hunger, fantasy, flickering old realities and a longing for enchantment may we find the way.

---

* From a story in *Long After Midnight,* a short story collection by Ray Bradbury.

THE MAGIC WORD...

Magic, like other fabulous words we use in this book, cannot be completely and succinctly defined, because it means so many different things. It both feels and looks different to everyone. Some people see it every day, some don't believe it exists at all.

For us, magic includes, but is not limited to: that which cannot be explained by logic or science; transformation through unseen energy; use of (super)natural forces; change and power. Magic can look like the incredible happening right before our eyes; shimmers and sparkles; disintegration, disappearance or reappearance; bubbles, flames, reflections and steam; glowing lights and bright colours. It can sound like voices unseen, the natural world acting in concert with our inner psychological processes. It can feel like strength from unknown sources; a spark of electricity; a fizz of wonder and awe; a state of flow; a warm feeling of contentment or pulse of unity.

Magic teaches us that things which seem to be impossible are possible. Things that have become separated, blocked or broken, can be re-joined, but often in unknowable, unseen ways, not by the standard cause-and-effect rules of science. Magic can imbue us with a sense of hope, empowerment, and perhaps help us to understand a little better the interconnected universe we inhabit. Magic is also a distinct way of participating in one's life and potentially influencing the direction in which we travel.

The awareness of an unseen world beyond our day-to-day existence is something all cultures have recognised in some way. It reminds us that not everything in this world is definable, concrete or absolute. Whether you believe or not, we live in a world that has always been fascinated by the promises and invitation that magic holds. We invite and offer up space within this book to find your own connections to the word, and your own way to magic.

WHAT IS A KITCHEN WITCH?

We come from bread and fire, from resourcefulness and intuition, from tinctures and time, from spiced cider and healing, and from long lines of sweet jellies shining in the sun. We come from the ordinary magic of ordinary lives. In kitchens around the world, we remember.

Molly Remer

A kitchen witch is one who celebrates the seasons of life through their kitchen. Who knows it to be a place of industry and sanctuary, confidence and caring, nurturing and healing. Whilst not a gendered term, throughout history and still today, the vast majority of those who identified as – or were accused of being – witches would have been women and this book is focused on female practitioners of kitchen witchery.

A witch is a woman of power and knowledge, her abilities were often feared and condemned by others, especially patriarchal powers that desired complete control over the minds and bodies of populations. This stain has stayed, and for many there is still fear and mistrust connected to this term, something we hope to dis-spell here together.

Many strands of cultural and spiritual heritage were, and are, carried in skilled hands by women and those who may have called themselves witches. This carrying was done through every craft of home and hearth, not just cooking but spinning, foraging, weaving, herb-craft, divination, song, prayer, and ritual, acts that have been lost through industrialisation and the imposition of Industrial Time.

The work of the kitchen witch is often to transform the inedible into the edible… "eye of newt" and "tongue of dog",* would be ways of slipping the least desirable cuts of meat into a pot, along with herbs and spices to make it both appetising and nourishing. She takes the roots, leaves and berries from the fields and hedges and prepares and preserves them, to feed and to heal. She intuits what is needed and learns to slip it in unseen, to disguise a bitter taste or unpalatable texture. She uses food and magic to transform. And has done so since the dawn of time when humans gathered and feasted together.

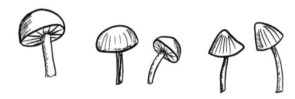

The kitchen witch works on many levels, often simultaneously, with purpose and intention. These are the main threads of kitchen witchcraft that we will be focusing on:

☾ **The literal:** the preparation of food

☾ **The metaphysical:** working with unseen energies such as the pull of sun and moon, the turn of the seasons

☾ **The metaphorical:** using ingredients for symbolic purposes

☾ **The medicinal:** using food to heal

☾ **The ritual:** using food in ritual and spell working

☾ **The ceremonial:** centring food at the heart of celebration and ceremony

☾ **The aesthetic and magical:** using food to enchant, bewitch and delight

* Used by Shakespeare's witches in *Macbeth* – interestingly they are actually pseudonyms for mustard seed and a plant called houndstongue, though real tongues, legs, eyes may well be used in cooking as well!

☾ **The alchemical:** using food as a medium of transformation.

The kitchen witch is usually not just a cook but also a herbalist, homemaker, artist, healer, crafter, grower, ritualist…her practice is diverse and multifaceted, but connected to food and the kitchen. She reminds us all that the ordinary arts of daily life have a magical quality: the alchemy of cooking, the herbal magic in your garden, and stories at your own hearth are to be valued and treasured. She reminds us that we are more powerful than we know. That our homes, hearths and bodies are the seats of that power. And that the magical can become part of daily life when the kitchen is (once again) considered a sacred space.

You may not have considered yourself to be a kitchen witch before. You may have heard or used the term hearth witch, cottage witch, green witch, or perhaps you have not had a name for what you do, or even considered it needed one. Certainly few of our mothers, aunts and grandmothers would have identified as witches.

One of the things that's exciting about being a witch in today's modern world is that there are numerous ways to be one, and no two witches will ever be the same.

Susan Tuttle, *Enchanted Living,* **Witch Issue**

After reading this book you might want to try on the term for size, step more publicly into this identity or stash it away as a treasured secret maybe, it's up to you. In whatever way you think of yourself today or ten years from now, however your practice and identity evolve and change, know yourself welcome here in our virtual kitchen.

This is how a few of our contributors understand the term 'kitchen witch':

To enjoy a little magic and enchantment in my home and kitchen is something I very much enjoy, and I am always learning more about how to bring the sacred onto my kitchen surfaces…

The more I research and write about witches, the more complex sometimes the idea of identifying as a witch can be. Hundreds of thousands of lives of (mainly) women were taken in many ways, they would have done anything to not be called 'witch'. What perhaps is the biggest luxury for me now is that when people ask if I am a witch, I can say I don't know, and my life does not hang in the balance of convincing people of that answer. And I can settle perfectly happily in a place of magic, enchantment and 'not-quite-knowing'. I like the possibilities within a world where I do not have all the answers. I can journey with curiosity and compassion, through long and ancient paths of foodways, ritual and folk magic that have laid deep rooted foundations for what we may call kitchen witchery today.

SARAH

Before starting to write this book I would not have publicly identified as a witch. It has been an identity that I have been edging up to and running from for well over twenty years, so I totally understand the fear involved for many in this identity. In the end what I call myself is less important than what I am drawn to and what feels most right to me in this world – and that is a personal connection to spirituality which is usually accessed through nature or ritual; a love of food and cooking, feeding others and eating together; a passion for the changing seasons, celebrating them through ceremony, food, gathering and crafting; a commitment to cyclical living; a deep connection to wild plants; a curiosity about healing beyond Western medicine; a fascination with the symbolic; a dedication to reclaiming the sacred feminine and women's culture. I have a shelf of books on witchcraft and several more on food and cooking. I also have a healthy disregard for the patriarchy. I think to most people this would define me as a witch. So I am (finally) claiming it – and stated it on the most recent census form for good measure! I don't think you can get much more public than adding it to the historical records… and writing a book on it!

A kitchen witch, for me, is someone who alchemises in the kitchen, often without even realising they are doing so. Someone who conjures magic through flavour, energy and creativity into the food, drink or medicine they are making. I am a kitchen witch most days – but more specifically when creating Moon Time Chocolates. I make most of my tinctures from foraged plants and organic vodka, and when making the chocolates I become a dancing creatress of herbal magic as I place drops of oils, spoons of tincture and sprinklings of powder into the mixes. This is my happy place.

Milly Watson Brown

I follow what some would call a syncretic Christian/Pagan path, which I would describe as Christian Animist, and so I have a rich and many layered wealth of tradition to draw on when I think about the term 'kitchen witch'. For me, the kitchen is the first altar and so a kitchen witch is someone who recognises that and seeks to weave a deeper relationship with food and cooking than the creation of nourishment only for the body. The kitchen witch also seeks to cook up nourishment for the soul.

Jacqueline Durban

I am a proud kitchen witch. For me, a kitchen witch is the true heart and soul of the home, a person who by their sheer command of the kitchen envelops everyone with that warm comforting glow.

Indra Roelants

I am a kitchen witch because I know no other way to be. There is help and hope and healing in a relationship with food, plants and herbs which understands them as pleasure, nourishment, medicine and transformational aids. We are composed of what we consume, and I have learned that the food we create has the power to help, heal, soothe and transform ourselves and others. My practice has been long in the making – from learning to bake with my grandmother, to the patient lessons of my mother's allotment. Food takes time, intention, care and balance: not too much rain, nor too much sun.

Alice Tarbuck

Ultimately what defines who a kitchen witch is, what she does, and whether in fact you are one is… you.

ONCE UPON A TIME...

Once upon a time there was a witch.

She lived in a house made of straw bales and red earth surrounded by thorns and oak trees.

She watched the world turn and studied all the mysteries she could, learning from crow and stone, moss and mushroom.

She followed hoof prints across steep hillsides and stony gullies and listened to lessons taught by wind and violet.

She lived in a forest, cocooned on a hilltop in a bowl of trees and rocks and sky.

She trusted in woodpeckers and deer, in moonrise over cedar trees, and in slow running river water.

She discovered the sacred in her own skin and knew secrets that are only found in being present to bear witness to the world as it weaves its poems before her eyes.

She learned stories and secrets from the berries and leaves and turtles and raccoons and she twined them all together into a cloak of power that encircled her with magic wherever she walked, and she walked often, simply for the joy of it.

Molly Remer

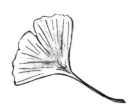
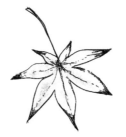
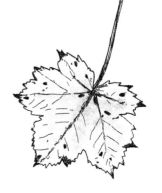

Kitchen Witch, Domestic Goddess, Housewife, Homemaker: Archetypes of Woman

Cooking is one of the strongest ceremonies for life. When recipes are put together, the kitchen is a laboratory involving air, fire, water and the earth. This is what gives value to humans and elevates their spiritual qualities.

Laura Esquivel

For too long, women were forced and cajoled into being the perfect housewife and homemaker, each isolated in their own individual home: obedient handmaidens to the patriarchal project by dint of the bodies they were born into. With any other form of creative expression or fulfilling paid work denied them, women learned to compete with each other over their domestic achievements: the most beautifully decorated house, best pie, prettiest dress, most accomplished children…

Our celebration of the kitchen witch is not a desire to revivify the 1950s aspiration of the Domestic Goddess or the Victorian "Angel of the House". These archetypes of idealised domestic femininity on which our mothers and grandmothers were raised are ones that most of us explicitly reject as disempowering to women. And yet they have seeded themselves somewhere in our unconscious expectations of 'how things should be'…how *we* should be if we are to be 'good' women. They are terms we – or others – measure ourselves against and often find ourselves failing. Or we actively rebel against them, dismissing all things domestic and taking on the mantle of the good feminist woman: high-achieving, hard-working, socially responsible, rejecting all things domestic. But in the mix of the rejection and rebellion, we have lost a primal sense of connection: to our homes, to our families of origin or creation, to what we eat, to ourselves, and to the natural world from which our food comes. We often find ourselves replacing care with frustration and resentment, feeling alienated from the place we call home and practices of belonging. We lose connection with each other in our busyness, exhaustion and competitiveness.

Interestingly, the term 'Domestic Goddess' points to a much earlier part of our history that has been occluded. A way of life that centred the sacred at the hearth, and honoured the divine feminine in daily life. The original domestic goddesses, deities of hearth and home – Demeter, Brigid, Vesta – were presences that would be prayed to, honoured and have offerings made to them in every home.

Before the 1950's vision of the Domestic Goddess was crafted, the role of homemaker was very different, as Shannon Hayes writes so persuasively in her book, *Radical Homemakers*. Pre-Industrial Revolution homes would have been reasonably self-sufficient for food, education, medicine, clothing and entertainment. This housewife was not a servant to the master of the house, nor a pathetic pretty thing, but a multifaceted productive creative human engaged with all aspects of crafting a life connected to both community and the natural world. She did not hold sole responsibility for her domestic sphere – instead work was shared: between multiple generations and members of the community.

We wholeheartedly agree with Seren Bertrand, in her book *Spirit Weavers* when she writes:

The deep alchemy of our times is for us to awaken our feminine magic – to quantum leap from housewife into a housewitch and magic weaver, tending the hearthside feminine churches. A home is wherever we live, whatever we love or tend, whatever supports, shelters, and nourishes us. No matter what our gender or work status, our home is our quantum womb and cathedral. Ultimately, our body is the most foundational home we have, inside the greater home of Earth.

Home is a powerful metaphor for a true center, a birthing place, and a destination we return to.

Housewifery at its most secret heart is the loving, tending of our Mother Earth and all of life. The secret truth of every tradition is that the greatest alchemists were always the housewives. Unnamed, silent, secret, spinning magic worlds across time. Weaving life together.

For us, kitchen witchery is an act of reclaiming…

☾ Reclaiming our ability to make magic and meaning in our daily lives.

☾ Reclaiming our hunger and appetites – nourishing our bodies and souls fully.

☾ Reclaiming our power to create, transform and heal.

☾ Reclaiming our sensory and sensual selves.

☾ Reclaiming daily ritual and our personal connection to the sacred.

☾ Reclaiming pride in our female lineage, skills, crafts and practices.

☾ Reclaiming our multiple heritages and identities.

☾ Reclaiming our role as beauty-makers and everyday artists.

☾ Reclaiming home as sacred space.

☾ Reclaiming our connection to the natural world, to wild foods and wild places, to picking and growing some of what we eat.

☾ Reclaiming our abilities of discernment and intuition.

☾ Reclaiming the vitality of community and connection.

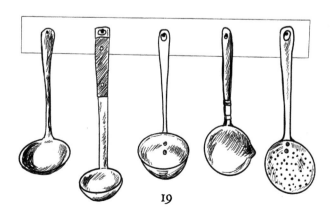

One of the simplest and most powerful ways to access the magic of the kitchen witch is to name and recognise her, in those around us and ourselves. This activates the archetype in our imaginations, bodies, minds and energy fields.

But what exactly is an archetype? It is a psychological blueprint. We all have many archetypes within us – Lover, Mother, Victim, Heroine, Fool, Princess, Teacher, Witch… energies, roles and ways of being and knowing ourselves in the world that come to the fore in certain situations. We have seen these archetypes embodied by many people in our lives, as well as in film, story and art.

When we choose to work with archetypes we can access their energy, associated skills, symbolism and rich human history. They can enhance and augment our own abilities, as well as offering a map for how we can inhabit the world in new-but-ancient ways. This is magic-making.

As we untangle these threads of what the witch has been perceived to be versus what she is, we can begin to leave behind fears and bias and can truly step into a place of magic, creativity and opportunity. So now, as we start in new ways and in new safety to embrace magical thinking, we can begin to envision what it might look and feel like to be a witch in the modern day.

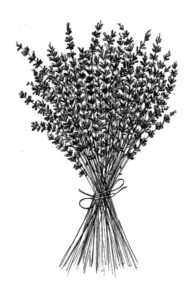

THE MODERN WITCH

Today the witch stands as one who is empowered, connected to the natural world and its processes, who engages other ways of seeing and knowing, who uses other technologies, and who has a personal connection to unseen realms. Her existence is an admission that science, technology, monotheism and capitalism do not hold all the answers they claim to. She fills the gap of something more, something else. She holds memories and echoes of the way things were, in the times before impending Armageddon. She holds the door open to a lost past that her ancestors were burned for. She has visions of worlds yet to come, and spells to help summon these. The kitchen witch reminds us that our kitchen, as the heart of our own domain, is a place where we can reclaim connection, power, healing and hope: where we can create new realities and share them with those we love.

After many generations of shame, silence and secrecy, witchcraft is experiencing a massive resurgence in popularity and visibility. And whilst the mushrooming of books on the topic is playing a large role in this, social media is undoubtedly at the root. Now instead of having to find a local coven or be an isolated solo practitioner, there is an accessible community of practitioners and resources available to you wherever in the world you live, at the touch of a button. Witches are publicly sharing what previously would have been private practice: altars, witchy bookstacks, gathered wild plants, spells, simmer pots, sacred circles, cats and crystals abound on Facebook, Instagram and blogs, educating, encouraging and inspiring others. Zoom celebrations intensified during lockdowns making ceremony on the internet a common way of practicing and connecting far flung witches together.

#witchyvibes and #witchcore are now fashionable, aspirational hashtags, inviting new folks into this ancient craft via an aesthetic. This visibility has taken away some of the fear around witchcraft for those tempted to dabble in the magical, opening up a wealth of ways to practice and identify.

But there is a cost too. The need to balance performance, superficiality and a need for acceptance and approval with deep ceremony, making sure that witchcraft is not done simply for likes or show, that practice is not surface level. The modern witchcraft aesthetic can mean that you can buy every crystal and prop and book online, and focus can go on the external, the aesthetic, not the inner alchemy. True magic cannot be captured with a camera: it is what goes on unseen, in the dark corners and hidden moments and shared celebrations.

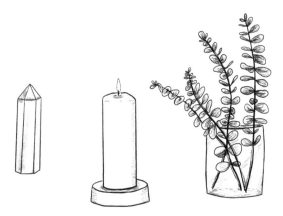

I have trouble sometimes reeling in my 'judgy' self when I see people 'doing yoga' for Instagram, because if they are posing for a photo they aren't really doing yoga at all – they are simply striking a pose. It can be similar for ceremony, spells, and ritual. In one sense they are always a performance: drawing the group together and inviting interaction. Or even on one's own, an action might be performed for or in honour of a deity. But performance for an audience on the internet is a little different – nevertheless still an art, and certainly can be of value. We can't tell you what is right or wrong for you, as always use intuition – are you connecting to what is going on around you... or are you seeking to 'look the part'?

SARAH

INITIATION

There is no monolith of knowledge or dogma that you must learn and repeat perfectly in order to claim the mantle of kitchen witch. Kitchen witchery is a dynamic, living, transformative practice. It changes you as you change it. It is rooted in need, hunger and desire.

Most of us have not been initiated to the art of kitchen witchery through an intact lineage of family practice. We are neither hereditary witches nor initiates. Just women making everyday magic, often unnoticed. We didn't learn these skills in Home Economics classes at school or from TV chefs. Instead, each of us is starting with scraps. Handfuls of family recipes, precious food memories, ideas from the internet, beloved fiction, the wisps of dreams and an intuitive desire to dive deeper into making magic come to life. We have continued family food traditions and made up some of our own. We have learned herb lore and foraging from books and friends, added magic by instinct not instruction.

We have both known many embodiments of the kitchen witch in our lives, though our guess is that none of them would identify as such.

For me (Lucy), the archetype of Kitchen Witch is most certainly an amalgamation of the women who have fed, nurtured and inspired me: my mother, stepmother and namesake grandmother, Darina Allen, Nigella Lawson, my friends Penny, Leigh and Laura. But it also includes fictional characters I have never met: Vianne Rocher from *Chocolat*, Tita from *Like Water for Chocolate*, Clara from *The Cook of Castamar*, the Owens sisters from *Practical Magic*, Willy Wonka… those who made love spells with herbs and chocolate, who could speak in the language of food and shift the destiny of others through the application of their magic.

As we reflect on what a kitchen witch is, at times we may begin to worry that it is a form of fantasy, but then we remember that fantasy is in fact an over-laying of the magic of the limitless mind on our material reality. Dreams, imagination, vision and ideas are brought into form through will, desire and action: this is at the root of all creation and transformation. This is at the root of magic. Little new is accomplished without the imagination. It is not lesser just because it has not yet taken form in this world. The imagination can bypass the inconveniences of time, space, economics and education. It is its own reality unto itself: the seed ground of a new material reality.

Some things can be both real and imaginary at the same time.

Joanne Harris, *Blackberry Wine*

There are also places where fantasy can get in the way of our embodying the Kitchen Witch: if we're waiting for the perfect home, kitchen, empty calendar, flying broom, big black cauldron, coven, spice rack or family set up. We must start where we are, with what we have, as we are. It is enough. More than enough.

THE CAULDRON

Double, double toil and trouble;
Fire burn and cauldron bubble.

William Shakespeare, *Macbeth*

The witch is usually associated with a bubbling cauldron. Names and ways of telling the story may change, but the magic of the kitchen witch has always been there bubbling away. The image of the wise/ terrifying woman cooking up magic in her big black pot, creating recipes of the esoteric at her hearth is timeless. All sorts of magics can come from the cooking pot.

The cauldron represents many things in folklore. As a symbol of the Mother Goddess, it symbolises the womb, nourishment, heat, regeneration, time, fate, transformation and creation. Cauldrons are also associated with Western alchemists: the containers within which the magic of transformation occurs – literally and metaphysically.

If you are ever in doubt about how you are using your energy or attention, a piece of advice that any witch would approve of would be: 'come back to your cauldron'. The cauldrons where we stir up our magic, where alchemy and transformation occur and where we can call our energy back home: take time to refill and refuel, to stir and reflect.

So allow yourself to seed your fantasy kitchen witch and her dream space in your real life. Find your heroines in fiction and reality. Pay homage to those you have learned from. Summon your personal kitchen spirits: these might be your mother or grandmother, the Goddess or archetype of Kitchen Witch. Ask for their blessings, guidance, support, wisdom and insight. Be playful. Take risks. Make space for whimsy and beauty. Allow yourself to be curious, to stretch and learn and make mistakes and try new things you might not like… just in case you do. Allow yourself to feel and follow your hunger and your intuition. Allow your practice to expand, to incorporate both your reality and your fantasy, so that you can embody more of your magic in your daily life, so that the world opens up further to you.

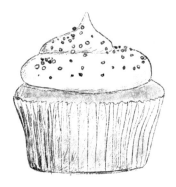

When I first read the words – the mystic cookfire – in Clarissa Pinkola Estés' seminal book, Women Who Run With the Wolves, *something woke up deep inside my heart. In her book, she writes about our inner Wild Woman: 'We may have forgotten her names, we may not answer when she calls ours, but in our bones we know her, we yearn toward her, we know she belongs to us and we to her.'*

We're able to 'taste' Wild Woman through flashes of inspiration. Often, we recognise her by seeing someone who has embraced this part of herself.

Clarissa writes: 'The longing comes when one realises one has given scant time to the mystic cookfire or to the dreamtime, too little to one's creative life, one's life work or one's true loves.'

The mystic cookfire, a place where we creatively daydream, should be woven into the life of every young girl. For in the hearth of the home we discover the foundations of nurturing ourselves and others.

Veronika Robinson, *The Mystic Cookfire*

MAGIC BOOKS

Many of us were first initiated to magic through the pages of a book. Kitchen magic is no different. Opening the cover of a cookery book can immediately transport us into other culinary worlds via the imagination: the kitchens, gardens, feasts and treats of others we have never met, conjuring sensory delight through word and image. They awaken the kitchen witch within through an imaginative journey into food, possibility, desire and delight… tasting fantasy and then bringing it to life. And unlike with fiction, a cookery book provides a recipe so that we can recreate the magic ourselves, giving practical guidance on new ways to combine ingredients, new methods, flavour combinations.

For many of us our most treasured recipe books are not the hardback tomes with stunning photographs by celebrity chefs, but the faded, dog-eared, handwritten, stained notebooks of mothers and grandmothers, the paperback covered in blobs of cake batter and marked with Post-it notes.

We sincerely hope that this book you hold in your hands now will be a treasured portal to the art of kitchen magic.

My grandmother Lucy died several years before I was born, leaving me her name and the memories of others. A biologist and educator by training, she was renowned for her culinary abilities. I have come to know her through her recipes…cooked by my parents and her friends. My stepmother found her recipe cards as we cleared their house after my grandfather's death. Handwritten in different coloured inks, on the back of old business stationary, her tried and tested recipes for coffee and walnut cake, tomato chutney, pithiviers cake and terrine emerged…some recipes so dated that they will never be recreated and others as ever-green and alive today as they were when she cooked them fifty years or more ago.

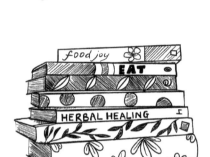

I have a lot of cookbooks, brightly coloured and fantastic, vintage and crumbling, all within which I find a form of escapism. All the beautiful recipes I will create one day, in a time of fuzzy future. Maybe it is the possibility of making them, on sunny days at elegant parties that very possibly won't ever happen.

Some recipes work out well, some much less so, I have a beautiful book of recipes to boost the mood, a very aesthetically pleasing book featuring two women embracing the mood-boosting properties of foods. On a particularly low day I was convinced making their sweet potato and salmon fishcakes would salvage my sorrows. It was a complicated recipe – too complicated for my delicate state – and I stood crying over the frying pan at the fish potato mush I had created. I think the lesson I have drawn from experiences like these is that kitchen time is not always, and doesn't always have to be, magical and joyful. But finding a little magic can encourage joy – and in time we can learn what works for us, and what doesn't.

COME INTO MY KITCHEN

We know of witches' kitchens from story books and films. But what does a modern kitchen witch's magical space look like? Welcome to our kitchens…

My kitchen has large south facing windows looking out onto the woods and the sea beyond. The sun streams through them in the mornings. There are herbs hanging from old wooden beams. A full set of shelves lined with organised jars of herbs and spices, their names written in sloping calligraphy, a cabinet of curiosities of artfully arranged shells, bones and dried seed heads, my treasured copper pans and an old-fashioned balance scale. Homemade potions in bottles for every bodily ailment, each beautifully labelled. In the corner, a wicker gathering basket, a besom broom that sweeps by itself and flies. The washing up is always magically done. The cat is curled up asleep in front of the warm Aga range. A cauldron is bubbling on top.

The long old wooden table is laid ready for afternoon tea. The room smells of gingerbread. A bunch of garden flowers on the table. Beautifully pressed napkins. A steaming pot of herb tea. A plate of warm scones fresh from the oven. A bowl of homemade strawberry jam and another of whipped cream light as a cloud. A stream of women seeking my wise council visit me here. We see spirits in the steam, read the future at the bottom of our rose painted china teacups, a love spell, a knowing, a…

This is my fantasy kitchen witch kitchen. Then there is my real kitchen…

In my current reality the table is half-covered in the debris of daily life and needs wiping. The peeling table-top that we painted together – a piece of plywood to cover the surface whilst the children were young – in a mishmash of styles and subjects including a poo emoji! There is a mountain of washing up stacked beside the sink waiting for me to tackle it. The oven is an unromantic electric fan oven. The cat has fleas and will hunt your ankles. We have no wooden beams – our home is less than two decades old, one of twenty cookie-cutter houses. The kitchen window looks onto a seven-foot-high breeze block wall on a housing estate, over which we have grown roses and honeysuckle which need pruning. There, in front of the kitchen window, is my herb garden, the first thing I created when we moved in. A half-moon of thyme, fennel, calendula, golden marjoram, feverfew and chives, it is overrun with mint and lemon balm, backed by bay.

The art on the walls of our kitchen reflects the seasons and our creativity… the kids' art and my own. The fridge is a modern-day family shrine, with photos of loved ones still here and long gone and improvised poetry spells with *Fridge Poetry* magnets. The windowsill is crowded with terracotta pots filled with herbs, flowering plants, and a jar of calendula oil that has been infusing for six months now. Last year's winter herb wreath hangs above paintbrushes in the cutlery drainer, alongside jars of this year's jams and chutneys, glowing in jewel colours, taking up counter space – some labelled, some not. There are letters waiting to be filed or replied to, and a pot full of pens that don't work. The cupboards are filled with pottery and glasses made by friends and family alongside Japanese bowls, and cheap items from Tesco and IKEA.

The herb and spice drawer (I have been meaning to clean and organise it since the first lockdown a couple of years ago now) is overflowing with glass bottles and jars. There is a strange smell, location and provenance unknown. The bin needs emptying… I add just one more thing to it, squashing the contents down, hoping someone else will empty it.

Laundry is airing on the radiator below the two overloaded cookery bookshelves… incantations of future food yet to be conjured. Floating shelves made by my husband are adorned with large plates made by my father, a family portrait by me, and birthday cards now several months old. A wooden dresser – the heart of any kitchen – is adorned with bowls of fresh and festering fruit, family photos, painted pebbles, clay models drying. Its drawers are stuffed with batteries, candles and playing cards, its cupboards bursting with art supplies.

Some days there are scones and homemade jam. (Though I may need to scrape the mould off the top of the jam and sniff it first to see if fermentation has hit in.) Other days all I have to offer is a pack of store-bought cookies. Some days the table is adorned with fresh flowers from the garden. Other days wilted ones with rancid water (perhaps that's the source of the smell!) But it rarely all comes together. Life, kids, executive dysfunction and exhaustion… in other words, reality, usually get in the way of my fantasy. But still I hold it in my mind's eye. Just as I hold the image of me as kitchen witch in my heart, even when reheating leftovers for dinner in the microwave, eaten in my pyjamas on the sofa, cat on lap, watching MasterChef on the TV.

The kitchen as the heart of the home, that cliché, that short sentence which conjures up images of smiling children, gathered around a wooden table, spoons in hand, eagerly awaiting the rather rotund mother, complete with apron and waving a large wooden ladle, ready to scoop oodles of thick stew out of a large steaming pot and straight into their bowls.

We all know it, we all picture it in our mind's eye, and we all have a small smile whilst doing so, the image transmitting an instant warmth and feeling of utter happiness and love.

The reality of course, is very different. Or is it? Replace the apron with a pair of jeans and the ladle might become a slotted spoon or even be absent all together, as the food is placed on the table and the children may help themselves or take turns serving each other and suddenly the image is very much the same.

A timeless snapshot of family life, of that daily ritual of feeding and eating. We cannot do without nourishment, be it physical or psychological. The sacred ritual of eating together, that is what makes the kitchen the heart of the home.

No matter who you are, how you are feeling, if you are ill or battling the raging hormone storms of life, one way or another we will end up back in the kitchen looking for comfort and love. But not just any comfort and love: that warm, loving mothering feeling only good food can bring.

Indra Roelants

Every morning I shuffle downstairs in my dressing gown and make a coffee for myself and a tea for my beloved. My kitchen is a mess. And I am always knocking mugs, spoons, and spices off the counters onto the floor and then silently blaming my partner because it's my job to cook and his job to do the washing up and put these offending items away – but more often than not they hang out on counters for days at a time. But really, it's also because I am a ludicrously messy cook and because I have terrible hand-eye coordination, and often toss things about carelessly. True story – in our last property there was pasta sauce on the ceiling, I'm still not sure how I managed it!

I have French doors in my little new-build house in the country that open onto a bed of rosemary and lavender. We (when I say we, my partner does almost all the work!) grow courgettes, strawberries, tomatoes, basil, thyme, rosemary, gooseberries, and figs in our garden. And I happily create chutneys, sauces, and pesto (recipe later!) from our glorious produce.

My dream kitchen would have a sofa in front of the doors so I could watch the rain on the garden. And cupboards full of beautiful jars of chillies and spices, and blue cupboard

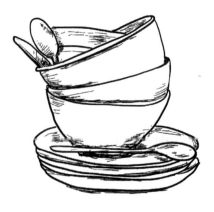

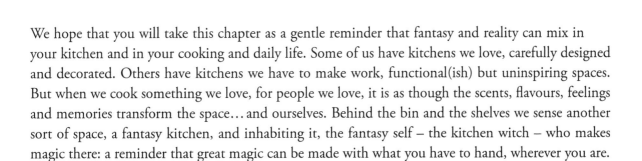

doors with shining copper handles and black marble countertops. (Our kitchen cupboard doors are actually white – my partner said they had to be white, better for reselling a house, god I hate being an adult!) And finally, I would like an art deco bar – with cocktail glasses of every shape, a hundred whiskies in shining bottles and A Nightingale Sang *in* Berkeley Square *on the gramophone…which I think places my fantasy kitchen somewhere between* Bewitched, The Great Gatsby *and the midnight margaritas of the Owens sisters.*

We hope that you will take this chapter as a gentle reminder that fantasy and reality can mix in your kitchen and in your cooking and daily life. Some of us have kitchens we love, carefully designed and decorated. Others have kitchens we have to make work, functional(ish) but uninspiring spaces. But when we cook something we love, for people we love, it is as though the scents, flavours, feelings and memories transform the space… and ourselves. Behind the bin and the shelves we sense another sort of space, a fantasy kitchen, and inhabiting it, the fantasy self – the kitchen witch – who makes magic there: a reminder that great magic can be made with what you have to hand, wherever you are.

The Kitchen Witch Emerges

The Kitchen Witch emerges with a waft of cinnamon, summoned up with the pestle and mortar crushing cardamom, with the harvesting of fresh rose petals. She emerges any time a pan bubbles or cranberries pop or the scent of melted chocolate or orange zest fills the air. She is there in the bubbling of yeast, the rising of dough, the whipping of egg whites or cream into billowing clouds, and the scent of freshly baked bread. She appears as spices crackle in hot oil and when boiling water is poured over fresh herbs in a teapot. She is there in a wonky birthday cake made with love or a stew for a grieving family. She is there as we gather the season's bounty from our gardens – a bunch of flowers to mark a birthday or a passing: roses for love, rosemary for remembrance. Her spirit is in the smell, sound and symbol, freed in the process of cooking, of transforming one thing into another. She is real here and now, in this strange modern world, if we choose to engage with her, if we allow her to awaken the dormant Kitchen Witch within us.

ON MEDITATION

While meditation is more commonly associated with yoga and Eastern religions, it is also a core part of magical practice. It is the starting point for other techniques and practices such as astral projection, manifestation, shamanism and 'hedge riding'. Meditation builds our ability to focus our attention and energetic awareness, both vital skills for the kitchen witch.

Meditation can also help us nurture and nourish ideas, intuition, imagination, empowerment, gratitude, calm and peace. Great transformation can happen in these moments, like in the cooking cauldron, before something new and beautiful emerges.

Meditations are not something you usually find in a cookbook, but we were keen to included them, as meditation is its own special form of transformative practice, of our consciousness and energetic bodies. We see the kitchen as a realm for all manner of magical practices, not just those involving food. Meditation is a tool we can all engage to connect to a sense of magic at times of celebration, seasonal shift and any time we feel inclined to take pause. Enhancing our skills of visualisation through meditation can allow the body and mind to relax, allowing us to journey through to places of intuition and knowing, creating space between busy thoughts and critical inner dialogues, so that magic and hope can shine in. Once more we return to that seeking: to satiate a hunger, to have faith in our own power of magic. Meditation can help feed that hunger and show us new pathways to magical experience and empowerment, creating a bridge between the fantasy kitchen witch and our daily lives.

How to Use the Meditations in this Book

Whether you use these meditations to lead a group or for your own personal practice, each journey will invite you to access your own deep inner knowing and sense of connection. They are perfect for reading aloud with a community, circle, coven or class, or you may wish to record the meditation and then listen to it.

How to Meditate

You can do meditation lying down, seated, or moving – while walking or cooking.

There are many forms of meditation, with similar practices spanning cultures – such as meditation to empty the mind completely of thoughts or to notice all sensations and emotion that arise without judgement. In this book I will be focusing on guided visualisations.

Meditation can be different each and every time: sometimes you may feel completely held in the experience, sometimes you may find yourself distracted and unable to settle. Try to be patient and practice non-judgement. This is a journey, it does not have to be 'perfect'.

Meditation is, as I so often say in my yoga classes, focus. That's it! It might be focus on the breath, but it can be on practices in your kitchen (also known as mindfulness) such as watching the steam rise from a cup of tea, stirring a pot, kneading bread, rolling pastry, watching bubbles rise, chopping vegetables…all these can be meditative practice, and a lovely way to – even just for a moment – let the stresses of the day fall away, and find our own little calm moment whilst gently stirring a pot, cup or cauldron…

KITCHEN WITCH MEDITATION

Today, we travel to the warmth of the hearth fire and the magical realm of the kitchen witch. To peek inside the kitchen of the witch is to glimpse into magic and into our past. This is a little journey to embrace the absolute joy to be found in the magic of hearth and home. Remembering the tinctures and balms our ancestors made from jewel-bright spices, shining fruits and emerald herbs. There is magic woven so intrinsically into the threads of drawing people home, feeding them and the laughter and healing to be found around the dining table. There's nothing quite like it.

So, take your time. Settle into your place of relaxation, taking a pause from the day. Letting the body and the mind settle.

You may already have found your mind wandering to the kitchen. It might be your own kitchen, the kitchen from your family home, or a special kitchen where you have felt safe and warm and nourished. It may even be a beautiful kitchen from imagination or a story. The room is aglow with light: candles, burning lanterns…and a hearth fire crackles in the centre of the room. The beautiful scent of wood smoke in the air. A smiling figure stands before a bubbling cauldron. Whirls of steam rise and dance. The potion within is one to heal and soothe…

Above the flames of the hearth, in the cauldron, story, history, and memory blend together, brought back to life in a sparkling moment: these create bubbles! And as these bubbles rise, they float around the room, and you see images within them. It might be a memory of meals shared with family. A romantic meal by candlelight, or one surrounded by laughter and friends. The cauldron is bubbling away, and more and more bubbles rise and float into the air. More and more memories dance in the light of the hearth fire. Allow yourself to see the bubbles. See the memories. See the joy that dances through this kitchen, and the magic you can sense here.

Pause

The dancing bubbles settle. You see the figure at the cauldron clearly for the first time, they are your fantasy of a kitchen witch. We've already mentioned in this book our fantasy kitchens, our ideal kitchen witch. Here you can envisage yours – is she glowing with health? Is she dressed as a perfect 1950s housewife with bright lipstick and bouncing skirts? Is she a forager with rosy cheeks? Is she a childhood memory of baking with your mother? Is she all these things?

Your fantasy kitchen witch hands you a bowl of the most delicious food. Take the bowl in your hands, it is warm and smells delicious. You and your friend at the cauldron sit side by side now, by the hearth fire, in companionable silence. The memories have nourished you. The food nourishes you now. The scent and the sights and the tastes of memory. And in this glowing warmth of the hearth fire, you become one – you and your fantasies of witch and kitchen blend together. Your hopes and dreams and memories, your notions, fancies and fripperies combine. You are allowed to be whimsical and romantic. You are allowed to be in love with your life. You are allowed to be enchanted by the magic of herbs and baking and syrup, simmers and seasons and sparkling wine! You are allowed to find great magic here.

Pause

As the time comes to leave this kitchen, know that your heart – the hearth within you – keeps these memories and joys safe. They are there waiting for whenever you need a little nourishment from memories that are sweet and magical and very precious.

RECLAIMING THE KITCHEN AS SACRED SPACE

When I was growing up and reading tales, lore, and myth, the heroes were always men leaving home, off to do something important, and even the heroine princesses ended up escaping from the palace, or from the tower where she was spinning gold. Housewives weren't heroic. In fact, you rarely ever read about what it takes to live a daily life: to tend your garden, grow your food, rear animals, build and maintain a house, clean, prepare, and cook food, raise children, and keep in good relations with yourself, the greater family, the village, and the larger community.

And you certainly never read or heard about the secret magic of domestic witchery – despite the fact that fairy tales were filled with witches stirring cauldrons over the stove or growing herbs, and that most magical fairy lore was set in the domestic realm and featured domestic duties.

Over time, I began to realize that I was looking far, far away for magical alchemists when all I had to do was look down at the place my feet were planted and the alembics of my own pots. In feminine magical tradition your home and body are the magnetic center that grows your power.

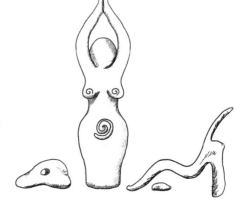

Seren Bertrand, *Spirit Weavers*

The idea that a kitchen is or can be a sacred space is not one that looms large in most people's minds. In mainstream culture sacred space is left to external buildings such as temples or churches.

We are sold the aspiration of a magazine-worthy bare kitchen, all gleaming empty surfaces, expensive appliances and hidden storage: a space that is – and should return to – neutral, with no sign of the seasons outside or of the life within its walls. Honouring the sacred, the magical in our kitchens is not something that is in any interior design guide.

Our culture has long associated cleanliness with moral goodness and left the unseen work for women's hands. It is for good reason that many of us have an uncomfortable relationship with cleaning: either being obsessive or avoidant.

I am a recovering perfectionist who is useless at housework. I have a hard time with accepting the chaos and mess of my house and not judging it as failure in my 'womanly' abilities to keep a clean home. My Kitchen Witch and 1950s Domestic Goddess archetypes do daily battle in my neurodivergent bodymind. I have to remind myself that the Kitchen Witch is there in the cobwebs and dark corners as well as the glistening jars of jam. She finds herself at home in shared confidences over cups of tea, whatever the state of the kitchen, despite what our culture tells us.

For most women the kitchen is intimately connected with endless drudgery and expectations. Cleaning is a moral obligation that hangs heavily and gendered on our shoulders. Much of the obsession with cleanliness has been to do with status, a way of occupying most women busy in a hamster-wheel of busy-work. We are judged by our ability as homemakers, as magical cleaning fairies whose labours must go unseen, from whose fingers come sparkling surfaces and billowing skirts come the waft of baking and comfort. Cleanliness as many of us were taught, is next to godliness. My goddess is thankfully not this god. My soul will not be judged by the gleam of my glassware.

For years I have struggled to invite people in – into my kitchen, my home, my heart – scared of rejection for this mess that I am not mistress of and what it says about me as a human.

Maintaining the illusion of no life in a home is a strange preoccupation. I chose to do other things with my time. Things I find more important. I have reclaimed my time from the drudgery of enforced perfection. Creativity comes first, not hoovering, in my home.

The kitchen witch is in a constant state of magic-making. Her space is part of that process. When we begin to see the kitchen as the creative and spiritual heart of the home, it is only natural that there be magical clutter and creative chaos much of the time, rather than the pristine 'show home' look we are made feel we should aspire to.

Having said that, we also love the occasional deep cleanse of a space to greet the new year, beloved visitors or to make space for a new project. At times like this we relish the throwing out of the old, the ceremonial sweeping away of dirt and dust, the ritual wiping away of the veneer of the past with lemon and water and lavender, polishing the windows to allow the light in.

The kitchen witch is aware of the impact of her practice of cleaning as well as cooking on the world. She does not seek to do battle with the unseen, she does not fear the menace of microbes, but knows them to be part of her kitchen culture, her own body. She seeks to harness their power to transform through fermentation. She seeks balance, not dominance. Living with. She does not clean to avoid emotional engagement or creativity, but cleans as part of her spiritual and emotional expression, cleaning and clearing not just the surfaces of her home, but the energetic realm too, to make space for magic.

THE BROOM

The broom is connected intimately to the witch. Much can be swept away with a broom. In the Italian folk tales of the Christmas witch *la Befana,* after she has gifted children of the house with treats, she uses her broom to sweep the floor, sweeping away the problems of the past year. In Russian lore, Baba Yaga flies across the sky in a mortar and pestle, with a broom made of silver birch to sweep away any trace of her path. To sweep can be a simple and powerful symbolic act to actively cast out that which we wish to let go of. Whilst sweeping, you may choose to set an intention as you move your broom, maybe you want to sweep trouble away, and out of the back door or clear a space for a warm welcome for all at your front door. Some use their besom broom for magical purposes such as cleansing and purification, and another broom to physically clean the floor. For others it may be one broom for both, after all every act of cleaning can have magical intent, and reminds us all our household tools can be special, without the need to buy anything new.

Creating Sacred Space

When we need to escape our surroundings, when it becomes normalized to seek solace and beauty everywhere but where we live, we forget the beauty of being, rooted as it is in the flux of process, of transformation.
Sabrina Scott, *Witchbody*

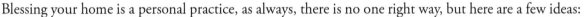

Your home is an extension of you. So, a house blessing can help welcome positive energy into both your space and your life and can be a way to imbue your home with what you wish to nurture in your life: love, peace, health, happiness… Many religions perform house blessings to bring harmony and prosperity to a home: Christian, Hindu, Islamic, Buddhist, Wiccan and Celtic cultures to name just a few. Meanwhile secular culture retains the idea in the concept of a housewarming party, bringing our friends' and families' energy into our new space, feasting to celebrate. Blessing your home is a personal practice, as always, there is no one right way, but here are a few ideas:

☾ You can do a house blessing when moving into a new home or when you want to bless a space in a new, purposeful way. You may do a house blessing when welcoming a new family member into it, after renovations, at the beginning of a new chapter of your life or as a regular occurrence on a special day, such as the old Scottish practice of saining (burning herbs in each room) the house on New Year's Day.

☾ Start with a little 'spring clean'. Clear clutter and wipe down surfaces. This may feel mundane, but it shows respect for the space and your possessions within it and helps connect you physically and energetically with your home.

☾ You may want to light candles, herb sticks or play music to set the tone.

☾ You may want to be in your house alone or with a group of friends or family.

☾ You may set intentions for each room or space of the home – especially relevant to the kitchen – do you wish to begin a healing journey with food in this space? Practice gratitude? Do you wish to repair rifts or reconnect at family dinners? Do you want to start a business from your dining table? Do you want to find joy in the kitchen? Speak these intentions aloud!

☾ Open windows and doors if you wish to release any old energy or memories. For new beginnings, open the windows facing east to let in a new dawn, and in the evening, windows on the west to release and let the sun set on old hurts.

☾ You can bring the blessing to a close in a room special to you or your intentions – for example: a nourishing feast in the kitchen, a healing soak in the tub in the bathroom, playing joyful music and dancing in the living room. (You could, in time, create a special intention ritual for every room in your home if you wish!)

Creating and Protecting Sacred Space

Jessica M. Starr

Sacred space is anywhere you feel safe, protected, and able to do deep work. You can approach creating sacred space in two ways. Fortifying and promoting the atmosphere you want and/or repelling or destroying the things you don't want.

We encourage and nurture the contact which we do want and we shield ourselves and our homes from unwanted contact, by having good magical hygiene, and by creating energetic barriers around our spaces. This looks like personal hygiene, housework, cleanliness, and perhaps a quirky taste in home decor. Many home protection practices are culturally specific.

The four steps, as I see them, are fundamentally the same.

Defining the boundary

The boundaries of our homes are usually visible and tangible. You may choose to work internally in the space, perhaps by walking into every room and looking at each wall. Or you may decide to walk around the perimeter of your land, noticing the edge, if you occupy a larger area.

Cleaning the space

Cleaning the space means getting rid of things, energies and physical items, which you don't want.

All of the elements can be cleansing, but water is the most cleansing of them all (which is why we use it to wash our bodies). Water which has been infused with a cleansing and protective Earth ally, such as salt, is excellent at clearing away energetic gunk.

You can also use smoke to cleanse your space. Smoke is excellent for space cleaning work as the air element means it spreads out and fills large areas. Certain herbs are good for banishing unwanted energies and others are great at inviting helpful energy into a space.

Light is banishing. The sun is exceptionally cleansing. Dark is magnetic, it draws things into a space. You can use light and darkness mindfully, alongside your intention, to invite supportive energies into your home.

Fill the space with what you want

This is something which it is helpful to pay attention to regularly. As well as cleansing and protecting your home, it is good practice to create a supportive environment for helpful energies and entities to dwell.

Salt and herbs can be dried and ground to a powder which can be used neat, sprinkled where you need them, or combined with water and added into washes. Or you might choose to use essential oils in room sprays, or pot-pourri, invoking the spirits of those plants and asking for their blessing and protection. Some witches like to keep spirit houses, such as skulls, hollow crystals or animal bones in jars, as places to home helpful spirits.

Reinforcing the boundary

You can place a shield around your house in the same way as you put one around your body, you just visualise it stretching out further, making a bubble over your home.

You can also use protective symbols to reinforce the boundary of your home. You can place symbols by tracing them in the air with your finger, or on a door with oil or water (or paint, when you are redecorating). You can also use physical depictions of these protective symbols, such as pentagrams, around your home. Traditionally used symbols of protection include The Eye of Horus, the Hamsa, five and six pointed stars, and all kinds of crosses.

Warding

Home and self protection is an area which can be overlooked. But an effectively warded home is the perfect space to craft other kinds of magic, whereas a poorly protected home can be the opposite. In a magical sense, wards are guards which are placed strategically to prevent entry of unwanted things into your sacred space. They can range from a small amulet worn by a person, preventing interference or entry into the physical or etheric body, or large like a lion statue placed at the entrance to a driveway of a stately home. (Or like gargoyles on churches or city gates etc. all of these are wards.)

Anything which is protective of you and your space can be a ward. Traditional wards include things like iron square-topped nails or railroad spikes (which make sense because they are pinning things down, preventing unwanted movement, cloves can also be used in this way as they are the same shape), horse shoes, statuary that is intimidating. All of these things have intrinsic warding characteristics due to the material, shape, or nature of the object. Less traditional, but also very effective wards, include things like house plants and charmed decorative items like paintings.

Wards are usually placed anywhere which could be an entry point for unfriendly Others. This is usually all the doors and windows, plus other possible breach points like chimneys and vents, and also in the roof space as there are usually very small gaps in the fabrication of homes which could be exploited. Walls, especially shared boundary walls, can be warded. Some people also use mirrors and other reflective surfaces on shared walls. Use your intuition to inform you where a ward would be best placed.

Walk around the boundary of your home and sense the energy as you go. Are there places which feel disturbed or hostile? It could serve you well to place a ward there. The same methods can be extended into your garden, if you have one. You just choose slightly different things to be out there. Hedgerow plants form excellent protective boundaries. For me that means mainly hawthorn, wild rose, elder and hazel. If you are asking for plant, animal, stone or other allies to assist you in the protection of your home (and this is pretty much always the case), it is polite to offer something in return for their service.

Altared Space

When we create sacred space we make a literal place for the mystery, the meaningful and magical. For many of us this is an altar space, something familiar to us from religions around the world. It is a dwelling place of the sacred and a reminder to us of the sacred each time we lay eyes on it.

Creating an altar may be a one-time thing, or something that you completely change with each festival or passing season, using cloths, candles and decorations in the colours of that time of year. It may include objects that represent the divine in traditional forms, such as a goddess figurine, as well as symbolic items, magical tools, photographs of loved ones and items from nature. We may choose to make it the place where we do spell work, say prayers or blessings, make offerings or charge items (in a sacred way – not our phones!) or it may just be a visual reminder of the season.

An altar doesn't just include things which reference or access the supernatural or divine such as a religious icon or sacred tool, but also the ancestral and spiritually meaningful. An old-fashioned kettle handed down from your grandmother, a bowl made by a family member, items rescued from a skip or house clearance… any items which hold emotional or magical charge and meaning to us beyond their practical usage.

This is how – and why – our coven of kitchen witches create altared space in their homes.

The kitchen is the beating heart of our home and so a lot of magic and ritual is centred in that space. It is especially a place for family magic, and I have our ancestor altar set up on a small low shelf near the stove. Everyone in the family leaves offerings of food and drink, and sometimes flowers or other lovely finds, on the altar space. When there is a family event we bring some cake and sometimes alcohol for our ancestors.

Jessica M. Starr

When I began making my own altars at home I made sure that they had a table of their own and they took up a central position. Now, my main seasonal altar is along one side of my kitchen worktop. At first this was a completely practical decision, that's where the space was, but now I find that I love having my altar there. My altar is my anchor, the place that I spin out from into the everyday world, and what better place to have it than in the kitchen? I also have a seasonal 'tree', made from willow twigs in a vase, on my kitchen worktop and decorate it for the seasons. I spend a lot of time in the kitchen, mostly making tea, and so I am reminded where my sacred centre is again and again through the day.

Jacqueline Durban

I came to creating altar spaces in my home not through witchcraft but anthroposophy, the philosophy of Rudolph Steiner. A Nature Table is a little altar space that Steiner schools and parents set up with coloured backdrops to mark the seasons, adorned with nature's bounty to reflect what is outside, and little fairy figures. It is truly magical. In time our Nature Table became a place where keys are stored, but also birds' nests, shells and pebbles found on walks. Now the children are teenagers we have garden flowers on the table or window sill, seasonal bunting over the mantelpiece and I have a personal altar in my bedroom.

This autumn I was tempted by the ease and bright colours of a fake autumn leaf wreath. But then remembered that it would be here for centuries after me. Whilst this autumn's leaves will be new soil by spring. Decorating your home with found things from nature goes directly against the "buy-buy" message of commercialism, it is another tiny act of rebellion against the capitalist system. It is an insistence upon value and meaning far beyond monetary cost.

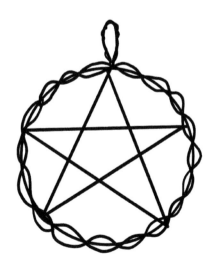

My kitchen is a sacred space because it is filled with the small acts of magic that live there and accumulate. There is the little purple witch, a gift from a dear friend, who is charged to watch over the stove and help ward off disaster. There are bells in the window, to keep ill forces out, and a watchful mask, popped on the wall, who is spoken to and blessed, and represents the house spirits.

It also houses all of the herbs I'm drying, or steeping in oil, or otherwise storing. I use bog-myrtle to ward off midgies in summer; clove syrup to drive away a lingering cough; fennel tincture or tea against stomach upsets. There's something cosy about it – everything jostling for space, always some project or another on the go. I think that is how I like a kitchen best – as the active centre of my home, always changing and in progress. Like magic, it transforms as it needs to.

Alice Tarbuck

RITUAL

Often our rituals are secret even from ourselves.
Daisy Johnson, "Ritual", *In the Kitchen*

Humans are creatures of ritual – from birth to death to how we make our morning coffee – we make meaning in our repeated acts of living. Our rituals are many and varied, from the elaborate and ceremonial to our everyday acts of sacredness that we use to ground and orient ourselves: the morning cup of tea, the bowl that must be used to serve a certain dish in, making a Christmas pudding together on Stir Up Sunday, the side dishes that must be replicated for Christmas dinner, where preparing the Brussels sprouts a different way feels genuinely as though it will knock the world off its axis.

We invite you to become aware of the rituals – large and small – that fill your days and years. Begin to honour them with greater awareness. And then, perhaps, add to them, as you feel called, more ceremonial rituals as you read through this book.

Sarah's Morning Coffee 'Good for the Blues'

One of my most simple (and essential) rituals is that of making coffee for my-self each morning. As I grind the beans, I listen to the whir of cogs, and crush a single cardamom pod in quiet prayer that my day will be filled with love and ease. The ground beans and crushed pod sit in their little paper nest above my tall mug; the water filters through slowly, and I can smell the coffee and the cardamom combining in rich dark liquid.

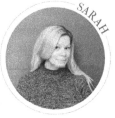

Originating in southern India, where it still grows wild, over a thousand years ago, traders carried cardamom along the spice routes from India and by the Vikings to Scandinavia, where it became very popular among the Finnish and Swedish in baking bread and pastries. Traditional Finnish cardamom bread, Pulla, is made with many cardamom seeds.

The pattern on my favourite blue mug (pictured here) is called Taika, a Finnish word for magic, and is inspired by folklore and fairy tales. It was a gift from my two best friends, fellow witches and yoga teachers, Trish and Tam. We had no idea of the provenance of this mug artwork when they gifted the mugs to me. But we'd been drinking from them for years as part of our weekly Friday coffee mornings in a lovely café in Bath – a chance to catch up with the world and city life and a ritual in itself.

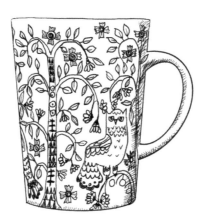

The best food rituals are, I think, communal and celebratory. Funeral buffets are among my favourite food rituals. We eat at funerals on behalf of ourselves, to reaffirm our livingness through the consumption of food, but we also eat on behalf of those who have passed, who can no longer participate in one of our most magical acts. To cook food for a funeral is to extend healing to those in suffering, to offer them physical comfort against emotional anguish, and to reinscribe our own animal bodies, which must eat to heal.

Alice Tarbuck

BLESSINGS

P rayers and blessings are often associated with the mainstream religion of our childhoods, the saying of grace before meals is something that many of us, having left religion behind, might feel resistant to. But blessings, protection spells, songs of praise and gratitude as well as offerings have been associated with humans and food production since the beginning of recorded history, in every culture. And not just when serving food but also when planting seeds, harvesting crops, brewing, fermenting and cooking.

Long ago, each act of food production, planting, harvesting, preserving and baking were done as ritual crafts, to the rhythm of women's songs, stories, blessings and prayers. Central to this was an honouring of the Earth Mother, household deities, spirits and ancestors – who in turn were thought to watch over the household, its health and harvest. All across the ancient world, women have carved the Goddess' sacred symbols onto pots and hearthstones and laid icons at home altars, made offerings to her as they gathered food from the fields and prepared it at the hearth.

We had some rather unrealistic dreams of sharing with you here many ancient songs and prayers said over food in sacred circles of women. We envisaged rhymes from medieval women, songs of Norse cooks, Celtic prayers to shoo away the fairy folk, maybe charms recited over bread and cakes to encourage them to rise… But we came back to Earth with a bump when we realised, of course, these songs of women, like much of women's domestic history and oral folk practices have been lost to time. Actual records of ancient prayers, rhymes and songs are not so easy to come by (though do ask your community elders… we would be honoured if you shared them with us, we'd love to hear of blessings passed though families and cultures.)

Modern day practices may be a prayer or blessing as we put a cake into the oven to bake, an offering of a libation when planting seeds, a blessing on the health and longevity of all who will eat the food. When sitting at the table, taking a moment to focus our minds, hearts and bodies with gratitude on the food and all the work of many hands it has taken to get it to our tables, the lives – vegetable and animal – that have been given so that we may eat, the sun, waters and earth for sustaining that life. It makes eating into a conscious act, stopping us in our tracks before we consume, bringing us together. A blessing may be said aloud or silently. It may be as simple as welcoming your guests with a toast or words of greeting. It may be sounding a ringing bowl, holding hands or a moment's silence.

These blessings are all little conscious acts to break the hypnotic spell of patriarchal consumerism and weave us back into awareness of the web of inter-belonging and awareness of the animate universe of which we are part.

MAGIC LESSONS

Everyday Magic

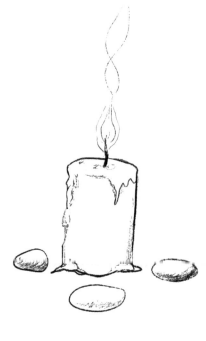

*It is a sacred assignment to rescue the crumbs of our souls
that have been kicked under the table by too much activity
and too little aloneness. To collect and kiss them all better.*

Sue Patton Thoele

It would be all too easy to add "make magic" to our never-ending to-do lists, making it a drudge and obligation, shaming ourselves with our failings for not celebrating every seasonal festival in a Pinterest-worthy way. But kitchen witchery is not about more doing, more making for its own sake. It is as much about finding and noticing magic, as making it. It is about the intention and process of inner and outer alchemy rather than finished products. It is about being present to witness magic in what we create, do and share in our kitchens. It is about coming home to ourselves.

Most of modern life is the opposite of magic. It tends to be energy sapping and juices us down to the bone, so that magic itself often feels like it is a childhood story out of reach from the grey haze of daily overwhelm. We may aspire to frolic through the dew drops collecting dandelions and spend afternoons gathering blackberries and turning them into jam. But then life happens. A child needs taking to a sports match, an animal needs to go to the vet, we're expected to work overtime, the oven breaks down, we have a cold…and our good intentions go out the window. We may long for a leisurely afternoon baking and end up frazzled on the road, grabbing a takeaway. We may slave away trying to make things magical and memorable for others, forgetting to include ourselves. We end up depleted, exhausted because we are trying to be the source of the magic, rather than working in harmony with it.

Our reawakening to the fantasy kitchen witch and her desires can make us disregard the limitations and reality of our very human selves and how much time, resources and energy we actually have to put into bringing this archetype to life in a world that does not support, encourage or even believe in her. We ask you to be mindful of this as you proceed.

Authentic magic-making looks different in the different seasons of our lives. We may have more time and drive when we are young and single. We may be more inspired when the children in our lives are young. Or we may find babies or work take us away from our kitchen witchery for a time. Or perhaps as children get older we find we have more energy to dedicate to our ritual practice, or medicine making for our community. As old age, illness or stresses compound we may find ourselves less able or desirous of elaborate rituals and celebrations. Perhaps we find a way to turn our kitchen witchery into a livelihood. Or perhaps doing so takes away the magic for us.

Not everything is – or has to be – magic. There are days and whole seasons where it may feel or seem unnecessary or impossible. Days where the kitchen is a place you would rather avoid. May we humbly suggest that these are in fact the times when magic is most needed…when you're feeling stressed, overwhelmed, harried or uninspired. When you have no time or desire to celebrate the seasons is probably when you most need to make a little space for sanctuary, intention for magic and connection. And it is also the time when the smallest spark of magic can make the biggest difference…if we will only open ourselves to the possibility. Picking a scented rose from the garden and taking a stretch in the sunshine. Watching rainbows cast in your kitchen from a sun catcher. Dropping a slice of lemon or lime into a cool glass of water and offering a prayer or blessing whilst you drink. Chopping a fresh sprig of herbs and breathing in their scent, marvelling at the green anointing your simple supper. A shared steaming cup of tea with a loved one as you pour your hearts out and

43

share your burdens. A bunch of seasonal flowers on the table, a cookie eaten fresh from the oven, a peach warm from the sun. A soothing scented simmer pot bubbling on your stovetop. Taking a mug of hot chocolate out to sit under the stars. It is about spotting moments for pleasure and connection and savouring them.

We invite you to explore what magic is for you – what it means, why it matters, what it looks like, what makes it happen, how your life is different if you choose to centre the magical. Feed your inner witch daily. Make your practice small and habitual, bring magic into the everyday, rather than reserving grand gestures solely for high days and holidays.

To create enchantment in our daily lives, to seek magic in the mundane is what we espouse. Not to live in a fantasy, but rather to bring elements of your fantasies to life. We share the building blocks – blessings, recipes and rituals – you can use to create your own everyday enchantment in the kitchen.

The kitchen is not the heart of the home. You are. Remember that.

PRACTICAL MAGIC

We have shared our opinion that magic can be found, and that everyday acts can hold magic: finding the enchantment in our day-to-day being is the real intention of this book. However, we appreciate that sometimes one may wish for practical pointers in how to make magic. Perhaps you need time to explore your intentions, and a ritual helps you clear your mind. Or maybe you want a spell with several stages to hold the attention and intentions of a group. You may have a precious free hour in your day and want to take a little time to dive into some magical work and would appreciate some suggestions.

With this in mind, we offer some spells and rituals over the course of the book, and very much encourage you to have confidence and trust in your own intuition to create your own. None of them are meticulously prescriptive because that is just not our way. Neither of us belong to any order or tradition, and we are not sharing specifically Wiccan or Druidic rites (there are many great books on these if that is what you seek).

We wanted to share spells and rituals that were most authentic to us, and that are open for you to weave in your own unique personality, energy and intentions. Finally, we have not mentioned deities but of course you are welcome to invite any you work with or are inspired by, to be present or watch over proceedings.

Starting Out, Building Skills

Some of us were taught the fundamentals of cooking and healing at home, others were not. Whether beginner or experienced kitchen witch, the path of learning new ways is the same.

First we become familiar with individual ingredients. We learn different ways to prepare each. We may learn where it grows, how to gather and preserve it. We learn its character and properties, the history of its usage and what cautions must be applied. In short, we befriend it.

Then we learn to combine one ingredient with another. We begin with well-known combinations, using the guidance of recipes or a teacher to build up confidence and working knowledge. This is where we begin to explore and understand alchemy, discovering how one ingredient impacts another... think parsley to take the heat from garlic and cleanse the breath, or sugar with rhubarb to counteract its sourness, or vinegar with baking soda to make a frothing leavening agent. Then, once we are well-practiced in the known ways, we can begin to explore new combinations, creating new ways.

We also begin to work on other levels: experimenting with the effects the different elements bring to a dish – the use of fire versus water or air – on texture, flavour and of course magically.

The next layer that can be added in is the ritual and symbolic, both in the making and in the serving, as well as the metaphysical, as we learn to cook in alignment with solar festivals, lunar times, or even your own body's cycles.

And finally, of course, the aesthetic, the magic of beauty. We are firm believers in flavour, nutritional value and ritual first... but if you can make it beautiful too, then all the senses and the imagination become engaged in the experience of beholding and consuming.

The remainder of this chapter will share some ways into magic-making if you are new to it... or wanting a little refresher!

Simple Magic

"Simplify, simplify, simplify," Lucy's grandmother always advised.

Simple magic is the often the most powerful.

Reflecting on the idea of a simple ritual, and simple magic, we were reminded of the herbal spell known also as a 'simple'.

A herbal 'simple' is a potion with just one ingredient. Essential oils are a form of a 'simple' that involve just one plant, as are herbal teas like mint or camomile. With these examples of simple magic we are shown that the idea of simple does not mean any less powerful. It is something that is uncomplicated and easily done. A singular focus – whether that be on a plant, herb, season or sun cycle – is ever more challenging in our busy world. So one may well argue that the simpler a spell is, the more powerful it is, because of that singular focus.

Sympathetic Magic

Sympathetic magic is a type of magic based on imitation or connection. It appears in similar forms throughout all cultures and eras: it seems almost innate to us as humans to find pattern and connection. Sympathetic magic is the belief that a person or object can be affected magically by actions performed towards something that represents them, such as work with dolls or poppets that represent real people.

The earliest forms of sympathetic magic may well be ancient treasures such as prehistoric cave drawings and carvings of the goddess. Archaeologists believe that many ancient cave paintings are the result of seeking successful hunts: the shaman or tribal elder would perform a ritual before a pursuit in which a successful trip is acted out, creating images of the hunters successfully killing their prey. Icons of the goddess may have been a way to seek her favour or blessing, offerings to the icon representing offerings to the goddess herself.

What we call 'the law of similarity' suggests very simply that 'like produces like'. We can use these ideas in magic if we wish to effect a change. Things that are connected can bring about similar effects. This idea is also the basis of the magical concept of 'correspondences'. For example, the element of fire can be represented by a collection of items that represent the energy of the Fire element such as sun images and fiery spices. They have the power to 'ignite' the body and psyche as fire does.

Sympathetic magic comes naturally to us if we let it. We instinctively know how to create groups and patterns from things found in the natural world through association of colour, form or qualities. For example, many of us could easily come up with ten items connected to the sun via association (flowers, animals, fruits, colours, candles, seasons, zodiac signs) with little or no prior magical knowledge. These would be just the kind of resources used in sympathetic magic. We will feature some correspondences and connected festivals after the recipes we share, but also encourage you to find your own connections, values, and memories, which are every bit as powerful. Cinnamon may warm us as a correspondence of fire and sun, which makes it popular for spells and ritual for prosperity and boosting of energy. But it may also remind you of your grandmother's baking or Christmas time. These are all valid in their value and in what they mean to you.

Instant Magic

Magic-making is often found or made in the details, in the little touches that we can do to make any meal – whether by ourselves, for a family dinner or for a large gathering – feel that bit more special. Most don't require planning, special skills or purchasing anything.

- ☾ Turn off the main light.

- ☾ Light a candle – or ten: tapered, pillar, floating, nightlights…

- ☾ Turn on fairy lights.

- ☾ Whisper some words of gratitude.

- ☾ Pick a small bunch of flowers and put them in a jam jar.

- ☾ Arrange your food on a beautiful serving plate – a tiered cake plate for sweets or afternoon tea, balti dishes for curries, a handpainted platter…

- ☾ Cut up a citrus fruit to eat or place a slice in a glass of water – the essential oils from the skin will brighten your day.

- ☾ Sift icing sugar onto a cake or cookie.

- ☾ Scatter edible petals on a dish.

- ☾ Serve an abundance of small dishes to give the feeling of a feast.

- ☾ Have a bowl of fresh fruit to decorate the space and enjoy.

- ☾ Put herbs, edible flowers or glitter into ice cube trays, fill with water and freeze.

- ☾ Sprinkle edible glitter on your dessert or even serve with a sparkler.

- ☾ Open a bottle of fizz – water, soft drink or champagne – bubbles are magical.

- ☾ Add a drizzle of olive oil to a savoury dish or a scattering of freshly chopped herbs.

- ☾ Polished special glasses or silverware twinkling in the light.

ALCHEMY OF FOOD AND COOKING

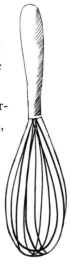

Cooking changes us. Eating does too. They are alchemical processes on every level: physical, emotional and spiritual. Harvesting, preparing and consuming foods weaves our stories together with the non-human world on a cellular level. We are essentially transformed by these acts. The kitchen witch remembers this.

Cooking and creating in the kitchen is an elemental alchemical journey: brewing, fermenting, leavening, transformation… Separate ingredients – some inedible on their own, like flour – come together with deft hands and practiced skill. Changes in temperature allow the yeast to grow, face the heat of the oven and be transformed. Water and flour mix, starches and proteins unravel, interlock and ferment. Each recipe has slight variations of how to combine, how long to rest, how to work the dough. From these basic ingredients come flat breads and fluted loaves, pie crusts – short and flaky – scones, cookies, cupcakes, pancakes, batter and even wallpaper paste!

The kitchen witch accepts as fact that when ingredients come together in the right way, at the right time, with the right knowledge, something far greater than the sum of their parts is produced.

Alchemy is, simply put, a process of transformation: this may be physical, symbolic, psychological, or magical. Alchemical practices concerned with the transmutation of matter, in particular with attempts to convert base metals into gold or find an elixir of eternal life, were present in many Eastern and Western cultures as an ancient forerunner of modern-day sciences like chemistry, medicine and psychotherapy. The art of alchemy has passed through the centuries from ancient Egypt, China and Arabia to Greece and Rome, and on to medieval Europe. The aims of the alchemists were to discover the medium of Eternal Youth and Health, the Stone of Knowledge or The Philosopher's Stone and the transmutation of metals: gold was the purest of all and most desired, and silver followed closely.

Sitting somewhere between magic and science, alchemists take something ordinary and from it create something extraordinary, sometimes in ways that cannot be explained by traditional science, hence it is often considered a magical practice. And because it is concerned with combining and creating, it is a word often used in modern parlance for cooking and kitchen witchery!

The Western elements of Earth, Water, Air, Fire are all present in the kitchen. Alchemy is occurring each time we brew a cup of tea – fire to heat the water, herbs from the earth, steam spiralling in the air. Each element plays its part, and we, the alchemist, the witch, orchestrate this amazing everyday magic.

Kitchen witches are first and foremost energy workers, creating physical energy from food, combining it with mental energy – memory, feeling, symbols – and using these tools to transform the bodies and consciousness and energy of those who partake in it, using season, setting, ritual, natural beauty, decoration and occasion to enhance the magic.

When working magically we consciously access the energy of the food and ingredients themselves, the latent Earth energy, the lifeforce held within, each in its own characteristic way: its defining smell, texture, flavours. Someone who knows how to work magic with food knows how to work with each of these defining elements, to compliment, contrast and enhance them.

Food is art and magic; it evokes emotion and colors memory, and in skilled hands, meals become greater than the sum of their ingredients.

Anthony Beal

Through cooking we learn about leaving time for bread to rise, and the conditions for yeast to thrive. We learn how to tenderise meat, harvest ripe fruits, preserve the season's goodness, to cleanse, to prepare, to share, to stretch, to aerate… each of the skills in the kitchen witch's repertoire has a psychological and spiritual adjunct – each element of manual labour holds a soul lesson too, if we are willing to slow down and recognise this. We bind and cut, we anoint with water or beaten egg, we banish air from jars to preserve the contents. Each of these is an act of witchcraft.

My mother was an alchemist in the kitchen

My mother was an alchemist of soul food.

It wasn't until after the death of my mother that I realised just how central food and the magic she wove into it was to my family's cohesion. Not just between our immediate family members, our kitchen was a hub for the wider community too. Her flare for food was the invisible glue that nourished and kept us all bonded. Without it our connection was broken. When she died her essence was gone and with it the magic she poured into it. She never wrote anything down, she created everything by eye. I wish I had paid more attention to how she wove her gift, but mother's food was just mother's food.

She was by all intents and purposes a witch, but she would never say that. To her creating a full banquet of food was just something that was a natural part of her. There was always food on the stove and people popping in each day to consume it. No one was ever turned away. Sundays together as a family brought a sense of normality. Even in the midst and heights of mind-blowing violence in the home, food was never neglected. Her gift of feeding us food from her homeland – Jamaica – made all relational chaos seem worthwhile. No matter what, the family would all get together at weekends for our ritual of breaking bread.

After my mother passed, I tried to carry on her traditions: but you can never recreate someone else's magic. Her gift carried a lot of responsibility too. Being the matriarch of a large family is a role that takes a lot of heart and one not easy to replicate. No one could make food like her. Her Friday fish was legendary. Her Saturday soup (Jamaican stew type dish) sublime. And her Sunday dinners reminiscent of the last supper. And the national dish of her homeland – a recipe I will share with you – brought the taste of feeling safe fully home to the body. When it was made you always knew that even if the greatest misdemeanour had taken place there would always be a truce.

There is something so potent in communal eating. I used to think as a child that my mother's pots were somehow magical, like the bag of Mary Poppins that had an endless supply of whatever was needed. Or greater yet, that she was a little like Jesus with his endless wine and fish. No matter how many people came through the door everyone got fed. Food brought a sense of community and consistency and there was something deeply loving and nourishing. Pitted against the transient nature of people coming and going, dishes became the healing balm in chaotic times, lovingly prepared with herbs from the garden. The rising familiar smells that permeated nostrils. The sounds of voices speaking my mother's tongue. My mother was an alchemist in the kitchen.

I am only just learning the gift my mother gave me through her love of food. As a child I thought I was missing out on something having all my food made from scratch. I wanted the convenience food my friends got to have. The fresh made juices and homemade sweet treats seemed primitive in comparison. Now they are deemed as trendy health foods, yet where she came from in the Caribbean to eat this way was the norm. My mother was way before her time it seemed. She brought with her all her wisdom about food and keeping the body clear and healthy.

I used to think my mother was cruel. Every day she would fill my brother and I with a spoonful of the foulest tasting oils to make our bones strong. Once a month she would deworm us with a bitter tea of boiled herbs. She would call it our flush out. Even our hot chocolate as children was now what I know to be grated cacao, but back then laced with nutmeg and cane sugar. I thought, why can't she just use the packet stuff like everyone else? So much of what she did seemed counter to health or enjoyment. How wrong could I have been. My mother was an alchemist in the kitchen.

I carry with me happy memories of the blood red sorrel she gave when she knew our energy was low. A drink to fortify the blood. Or the pots of twigs she would brew to bring down a fever. Or the liquorice root to clean our teeth. And the raw sugar cane to chew as a sweet treat. And her use of the whole coconut from its waters to its flesh. Watching my father chop them open skilfully with his machete and wondering who would get the first drink. To watching mother grate and chop its flesh to make an abundance of coconut drops, that would last for weeks. All things I took for granted. All things I abandoned in my teenage years as fast as I could. All things that have now become things I long for. I threw the baby out with the bath water. It seems so silly to me now that I wanted the fast-food my friends could have and not the food of my ancestors. I would do anything to have just one morsel of her cuisine and the nourishment of her soulful knowhow.

Coco Oya Cienna Rey

FOOD CULTURES

EATING TOGETHER

Food is a bridge to community.

Julia Turshen

Since our ancient ancestors first gathered together around burning fires in the earliest of communities, feasting has brought together friends, family and loved ones with spirits, gods, memory, ritual and magic. As we look back to our earliest ancient civilisations, food magic was considered powerful indeed. Religion and magic were all interwoven as the food was made and offered for deities by priestesses, herbs and intoxicating beverages were consumed by oracles and seers and everyday rituals were used to seek blessing at families' hearths.

Food connects us to both our physical bodies and our feelings. In most books featuring food magic enchanted food brings passion – be it lust, tears or truth – to the surface. Good food makes us feel deeply. Shared meals at special times fill more than just our bellies, but our memories and hearts. Food is often connected to companionship, the root of the word meaning 'one you share bread with'. Some of us live in busy house-shares, of family and friends, whilst many of us live without other humans. But that does not mean we are alone. Most witches have other companions: pets, wild animals, plants, stones, spirits of loved ones who have passed over, treasured libraries, visiting friends that shift the energy of the space and enrich it.

I am lucky to belong to what we describe in shorthand as Food Group, an off shoot of our Women's Group. We meet at each of the eight Pagan/Celtic festival of the Wheel of the Year. Each time one of the women hosts and cooks the main savoury dish and everyone else brings a side dish, either sweet or savoury. Each meal is seasonal, and the ingredients as local as possible. Each time foods are brought that many of us have never tried: a new ferment or pickle, a new foraged ingredient, a traditional recipe. Together we have tried: laverbread, bannocks, pickled black walnuts, orange wine, many wild greens, gorse kombucha... We feast and then we share music, poetry, a blessing, a passage from a book on traditions or a craft activity connected to the season or festival. We leave nourished on every level with fine food, new ideas, friendship and connection to the season and our land.

LUCY

A Culture of Food

In the kitchen, memories live in the body, just under the skin and under the tongue. Scents and residues from childhood rub off on our hands.

Nina Mingya Powles, "Steam" in *In the Kitchen*

What we think is good to eat, how it should be prepared and seasoned, when it should be eaten, by whom, how much and with whom, these are the cultural threads of food that define us and make each of our approaches to cooking – and food magic – unique. Our kitchen witch DNA is woven from all the cultures that combined to create us: the family cultures of parents, grandparents and other influential adults, the cultures in which we grew up, that in turn were shaped by climate, history, economics, religion, war, as well as trends and fashions. As individuals, cultures, a species, we are made of ferment and foment. The threads of our beings are woven from many cultures.

Our histories – culinary and magical – are shaped by cultural exchange and colonisation. By sacred sharing and forced suffering. We are often led to understand culture as fixed and singular, with traditions that must be rigidly recreated, otherwise the spell of reality and harmony will be broken. But culture is by nature creative, dynamic, ever-evolving. Often it is in reweaving the threads of the old that greater harmony and authenticity are found. As kitchen witches we learn to move away from force and towards consent and flow, co-creating with, exchanging with, working with... in endless experimentation.

We come from cultures and we also *are* cultures. We inhabit a space within complex cultures of species working together. We are host to a beautiful feast within and on our bodies – beneficial bacteria, viruses and fungi interacting and consuming us. We are co-evolving together. As kitchen witches we remember on the deepest level that we are what we eat, and so we begin to nourish our microbiomes with wild foods carefully gathered and fermented foods lovingly tended. Cultures within cultures within cultures. We remember it is our job to tend, nurture and co-create them.

When we learn to see the world with magical eyes, we begin to uncentre ourselves, as individuals and a species. We learn to leave space and give thanks for unseen interactions. We become aware of the magic at work within us as well as the magic we work. We know ourselves – at last, at last – as vital co-creators of culture.

THE COLONISATION OF FOOD

I heard a talk recently about the colonisation of food, in particular the herbs and spices of the Asian and Caribbean islands and how the esoteric deeper wisdom was lost when it was brought over to the West. The skill of how they synergised and blended together was discarded. Information about their flavour enhancing qualities deemed more important that the depths of their healing properties. A loss of the union between the dance of the masculine and feminine traits found in our food. It was in the combining of certain herbs and spices that my mother's food took on a whole different dimension. It was never just about flavour enhancement, she always desired to nourish those around her with the deeper thing.

When we don't honour the essence of food. When we don't give kudos to its deeper truths, they become hollow substances and discord is created in the body. We lose the richness of all it has to offer. We lose our connection to dirt and soil and Earth. We lose our connection to The Mother. We are a part of nature there is no getting away from that and when we allow ourselves to remember this, we can restore our connection to her. We live in a world where we are hungry for the mother. Hungry for the depth of nourishing connection that feeds the soul. This was the gift of my mother's food. She was always leading us back to the sacredness of food and the power it had to heal all discord. Let food be thy medicine was her ethos. Her way of loving was through her food. Food filled with love is a healing medicine in and of itself.

I had the best of both cultures. Food from the earth and ground that I learnt to fall in love with without knowing its history. And food that was native to this land. Both I appreciate on a deeper level. Knowing some of its journey from Caribbean village farms, to bustling towns, to overseas and British streets, fills me with delight. Mangos, avocados, cocoa…foods that are now plentiful on British shores which were the staples from my childhood now connect me back to the love of my mother.

Coco Oya Ciena Rey

Cooking to Comfort, Cooking to Heal

A few hundred years ago there were no differences between magic and medicine.

Joanne Harris, *Blackberry Wine*

When we are unwell we often lose our appetites not only for food but our hunger for anything that usually brings us joy. Confined to bed we lose connection with the natural world, and often to our own souls as our ability to engage in the practices we love falls away. Beyond the medicines that come in bottles and pills, it is often what is brought to us on a tray to our sick room, that invites us back to being fully alive, reminding us of the magic that lies within and without.

The ability of food to heal on every level – from providing needed nutrients to soothing the soul – has been abandoned by the wayside of Western medicine. The kitchen witch reclaims the healing magic of food and the ancient understanding of medicine to heal both body and soul.

Medicine is real food, good dirt, a hug or listening ear, the bird songs, a fire, clean air, strong winds, good water, a story from someone who's walked a different life than your own, ceremony, songs, and rituals that remind us of who we are, old stories from elders, imaginative stories from children are all medicine that we need at this time to integrate and cultivate and nourish, to be the ones to support the great changes of our times and ReGenerate hope for all of our children's children's children yet to come...

Amy Rebekah

The following reflections from our coven of kitchen witches highlights the healing qualities of food and its use to communicate what we cannot always say with words.

Healing Comfort Foods

In my community of foodie folk and witchy ones, there is a culture of gifting each other with food magic: baby aloe vera plants, scobys and kefir grains, sourdough starters, herb cuttings, extra veggie plants, chicken stock when sick, nurturing meals on births or bereavement, garden flowers for birthdays, homemade cakes, chutneys, jams or drinks, a bumper apple harvest or a great day's fishing... This is how we show love in our community: we come bearing food, it is our currency of care.

It is a care I extend to my family and myself as well.

Cooking a pot of soup after a couple of weeks of illness and feeling unlike eating reminds me of the magic of food. Softening finely chopped onions and garlic in butter, adding in diced potato, a pint of chicken stock to nourish, the bubbling pot, stirring with a wooden spoon, steam rising. When the potatoes are soft, plunging in chopped locally foraged watercress, packed with C and B vitamins for my immune system. A glug of cream, sea salt and black pepper and blend. Served in bowl made by my father. Nourishment for body and soul.

A mug of steaming ginger tea cupped in my hands sipped slowly to ease a migraine.

Rice pudding, plump grains of rice baked slowly in sweetened milk and cream, grated with warming nutmeg and curls of fresh lemon peel to ease a tender stomach or heart.

Frying up a paste of garlic, onion and ginger to boost the immune system, turmeric as an anti-inflammatory, cinnamon to warm, cardamom to soothe, black pepper to stimulate, stirring in red lentils, adding in tomatoes and coconut milk, gently simmering. A hearty healing dahl, topped with dark fried onions, cumin and fennel seeds for digestion popped in hot oil.

Miso soup, rich umami broth with floating treasures of wakame seaweed and spring onion to nourish and soothe.

A roast chicken with tarragon cream sauce and crisp roast potatoes eaten with my family, seasoned with the week's news, leftovers eaten greedily with fingers when clearing the table.

Hot donuts dipped in thick hot chocolate to warm us after a family snowball fight.

These are some of the dishes I return to, to comfort and nourish, to bring me back to myself, to heal my body, to comfort those I love. Each of the processes is familiar and soothing, so familiar as to no longer need recourse to a recipe. Each of the ingredients are added with knowledge of what they will do to body and soul. Making them is a prayer, a ritual, a way of coming back to life.

How can cut up fruit mean you are loved?

When I was growing up, I rarely had outward expressions of love. Love is often a complicated emotion in migrant households, it does not always translate to the words "I love you". For many migrants, including my parents, their emotions came second to their drive to make a life for themselves in a foreign country so that their children could live a life they had dreamt of — filled with opportunities and chances to excel.

But that is not to say that I was short on love. My parents show love in a different way. Whether it is the incessant calls if you are *five minutes late (they cared for you so much that they could not rationalise a bus being delayed). Or the way my mum would give me endless Tupperware boxes filled with curries and dhal to freeze and eat when I miss home. My fondest memory of my mum showing me love is a bowl full of fruit cut up. That bowl of fruit, usually whatever was in season, was a symbol of my mum's understanding, care and love regardless of what I was going through. We never shared deep meaningful conversations, but the peeled, deseeded, and pitted fruits were the only exchange I needed to know that I was loved. Whenever I feel down, an act of love that I do for myself is recreate that small bowl of fruit for myself to sit down and enjoy. It never fails to make me feel held in a way I struggle to describe.*

Khyati Patel

For many of us, what we associate with home cooking is the expression of love and nurturance of those who cared for us as we grew. For others a lack of food was associated with a lack of care.

Part of the healing journey for many of us is learning to fill the gaps we experienced as children in healthy ways. Beginning to fill the spaces where love and care was lacking in ways that do not damage or punish our bodies: moving away from binging or purging, from addictions to sugar or alcohol, towards kinder loving ways of dealing with hunger, hurt, grief, anger and loneliness. Filling the gaps with real magic and joy, care and kindness, not artificial quick fixes.

Sometimes it is as simple as choosing to make a fruit plate for yourself. Choosing fruit over candy. Cutting it up with love. Serving it on a nice plate. Taking time to savour it in the sun. Treating yourself as a beloved child, a welcome guest at your own table.

RECLAIMING WILDNESS

"There is a wild one calling you by name
In your most inconvenient moments.
Trust her whisper can reach through the walls of your domestic life
Arriving in your dreams
I commend you for not running at first
Wild and naked out of your life to meet her…
But eventually you will."

Marya Stark, "Bone by Bone"

One of the core threads of witchcraft and magic is the call back to a different relationship with wildness – wild nature and our own wild natures. Witchcraft is a reclaiming of the knowledge that there is a livingness beneath the things of our daily lives that we can connect to – a wild mystery at the heart of all things that the modern world seems to want to domesticate, ignore or destroy. The wildness is calling insistently. Our inner witches hear it as a call back home to ourselves. A call to magical belonging. We rediscover the magic of finding our niche in an interconnected ecosystem. We relearn the art of lying dormant, knowing that the time of blossom and fruit will come.

When I make food using foraged plants I find them inherently healing, both because they are full of vitality and because they help to connect us back into the land. They are where I find my true energy work lies. It creates a breathing out of long-held tension and often our healing really is in remembering to breathe.

Jacqueline Durban

What is the wild? It is life on its own terms – undomesticated, untampered with, life growing where it will, as it wills. Life that is chaotic, untamed, uncontained, both abundant and effusive, as well as rare and hidden. Elemental and interconnected. Untended except by the Earth and her other creatures. Life without bounds. Life that follows the cycles of nature, its own innate patterns and rhythms, unbeholden to clock or calendar.

How can we rewild our lives through our kitchens? This book is packed full of suggestions. By foraging and preparing wild foods, growing plants on our windowsills, tending jars of ferments filled with bubbling living cultures, using natural cleaning products, letting our cooking follow the seasons and cycles, composting our waste, using water mindfully. In our gardens we can let in the wild edges, leaving areas unmown, making space for the weeds and wild ones, not spraying or using artificial fertilisers but compost and manure, planting native species, nurturing plants for our pollinators, sharing our space with other creatures – providing places for birds to nest, hedgehogs to hibernate and birds to feed on pollen, bugs and berries, controlling invasive non-native species and of course foraging through the seasons.

The Flavors of a Living Year

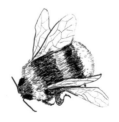

March tastes of wild violet
And chickweed.
April of plum blossom
And redbud flower.
May is flavored with morel
And dandelion.

June brings raspberries
To rest against the tongue
And July offers blackberries
With brief tastes of wild blueberry
In between.
In August,
Chanterelles and black trumpet
Mushrooms grace
Our mouths with glee
And in September
It is the flavor of puffballs
That we seek.
October tastes like persimmon,
Soft and orange.
November smells of cinnamon
And holds hints of hickory
And pecan.
December, ah, December
Tastes like frost flowers,
Cool curls of ice and dittany ghosts,
Dissolving swiftly on the tongue.
January is the flavor
Of snow ice cream,
Vanilla and snowflakes,
While February is spiced with persistence
The taste of cedar smoke and icicle.
Then we find the wheel has turned
And it is March once more,
Wild violets by the woodpile,
Stars of chickweed in the grass.

Molly Remer

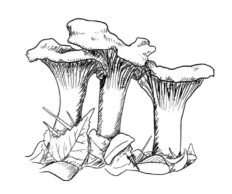

WILD SIGNS AND STAR PATHS

Let's start by going back to the very beginning – women and wild food. Because once upon a time all food was wild – and it was the women who gathered it. And from harvest to preparation to consumption, no aspect of food production was left untouched by magical ritual. Many ecofeminists see the oppression of women and the exploitation of nature as fundamentally connected, but because the banning of magic, the subjugation of women, the domination of the Earth – and the capitalist overtaking of food production – all went hand in hand, I see food magic as an important site for ecofeminist intervention.

Danielle Prohom Olson, "Ecofeminism & Ancestral Skills & The Reclamation of Food Magic", *Gather Victoria*

O ur hunter-gatherer ancestors were people in tune with the Earth, stars, and seasons who would, in time, create settlements, cultivate crops, and domesticate animals. Knowledge of the weather and seasons was the foundation of our survival: watching and celebrating the sun's set and rise; snows and frosts melting; green shoots appearing; animals giving birth and giving milk; crops ripening. Traditions, rituals and offerings grew up around these celestial, agricultural and seasonal cycles. They became special and sacred occasions, marked by the ritual preparation and consumption of food. To come together in feasts is part of our very earliest communal acts, from the dawn of human society. Festivals were feast times and a break from work and routines. Celebrations of gratitude throughout the year brought communities together to eat, drink and make merry; they were also times for reverence, reflection and ritual.

Sometimes the most powerful magic is the simplest, as simple as a rising and setting sun. The sun, its power and its cycles are central to our survival as a species and the growing of food. It is no wonder that it has been so carefully observed, celebrated, and formed a central part of most religious and magical traditions.

As the earliest gatherers, women observed the course of the seasons and weather, and many would become skilled in predicting their course and patterns. (The superstition that witches could raise a storm was far more likely to be their real ability to predict one.) Foreseeing forthcoming changes, weather, family fortunes and health, was a practised skill. One once possessed by all rural folks. But you can practice it again and learn to read the seasons, the weather, animals and nature.

Part of my mother's legacy was to teach me how to talk to plants as a way of unlocking the stored information within them. This was another way of imprinting their essence into the body long before they hit the plate. She taught me that plants would offer up their magic as silent whispers on an energetic level. Their wisdom seeping into the psyche revealing how they should be used or ingested. You would often find my mother singing or talking to her plants and apologising if she had neglected them in any way. This synergistic relationship between foliage and human could be felt in the ether and brought with it an awareness of our belonging to all life. Earth grows things that let us to get to know her and ourselves in greater detail if you allow.

So much of the wisdom of our plants and their medicine has been labelled irrelevant. Yet as we evolve there will come a time when our relationship to food will become much deeper. We will be taken back to the core root knowing that our food comes from living things and can feed and nourish the soul.

Coco Oya Ciena Rey

The namesake of this section, the book *Wild Signs and Star Paths* by naturalist Tristan Gooley, reminds us that awareness of the natural world can allow us to sense when changes will occur, from crops and weather to animal migration. But we have become so distanced from this way of experiencing our environment – and climate change is disrupting the predictability of these cycles – that it may initially seem impossible or esoteric. We can all reclaim this ability to connect, see and read the rhythms of the natural world, each turn of the wheel. To do so helps to imbue us with a deep sense of belonging – an experience often missing from our lives as modern humans when we live on, rather than in, the Earth.

The process of planting, growing (or foraging, or buying), and consuming food is an amazing cyclical journey. Seeds that are planted grow and ripen to fruits that might be offered to deities or consumed with gratitude at the altar of your own dining table. Remembering this magic process as you turn inward and reflect upon growth, abundance and gratitude can be special and powerful.

The kitchen witch is aware of the rhythms around her and works with them, anticipating when there will be times of abundance and scarcity, planning for them when she can, ritualising the thresholds, peaks and passings, helping to make ways to travel together through them, creating a narrative and memories with and through food and ceremony.

THE LIVING YEAR

To visualise the year in circular form is an ancient (and wonderful) act. Perhaps the most widely known circle pattern are the four points of winter, spring, summer and autumn. A wheel of light from the darkest days of winter, moving into the fresh green growth of spring and bright sun of summer before the golden days and leaves of autumn roll around and nestle once more into the cold and dark of winter. This wheel may be studded with glorious seasonal festivals, which can guide us both as individuals and communities, gifting a rhythm to lives and years.

The ritual year and cycle of celebration varies from county to county, nation to nation and family to family. Whilst we will be using the pagan/Wiccan/Celtic Wheel of the Year as a basis for the second part of this book – drawing on our own Norse, Anglo Saxon, Gaelic and Celtic heritage – we expand far beyond its confines to include a wealth of festivals that we find great joy in, from Bonfire Night to cherry blossom festivals and we invite you to do the same, weaving in the festivals from your own family or cultural traditions.

There are other shorter cycles to weave into our practice that we often overlook: the cycle of the week – Friday night takeaway, week-day packed lunches, the Sunday roast… Also the menstrual cycle, the ebb and flow of energy, rising towards ovulation, and descending as menstruation approaches, leading to more energy, desire to be in the kitchen, a need for comforting, warming foods as our period approaches, the use of herbal teas to soothe cramps, the increased desire for carbohydrate-rich food, and of course chocolate. We work real magic in our kitchens and lives when we make a regular practice of tuning into these inner and outer cycles.

WHEEL OF THE YEAR MEDITATION

Close your eyes and relax as we settle and breathe.

Let us visualise the circle of the year – we may see fields laid before us where the change in seasons can be clearly seen as the days pass, or a grand spiral labyrinth where the year's changes can be seen all at once. Perhaps we watch over this place, or stand within it.

Take a pause to see and feel the unique magic of each season:

☾ We start in winter slumber, dark, icy, cold, dormant, and restful in stillness. There is a quiet here that calms you, invites you to pause, and exhale a frosted breath. The Earth is paused, frozen for a moment in time. But a glow from the sun is just visible on the horizon, distant, but present.

☾ Dawn breaks and we begin to stretch into spring light and warmth like green shoots and flowers. You can feel a sparkling freshness, like morning dew. You can feel it in the air, crisp and bright.

☾ The sun rises high in the sky and you dance into bright sunlight. Birds swoop and sing in bright blue skies, you can smell sumptuous roses, honeysuckle and lavender in glorious scent and colour. A haze of heat shimmers over golden fields and beaches.

☾ See now, in your mind's eye, nuts, apples, browning golden leaves that drift and fall to the earth, golden sunlight glowing through trees as it sinks towards the horizon and bonfires burning with scents of smoke, roasting foods and fireworks.

☾ Now, gently, back to darkness, a rest and quiet fills the circle. Repeated through life, the years turn, but also each day, as we rise and stretch and dance into full light, settle down for evening and finally back to the dark rest of night.

See this cycle, see the changes, each day, each year, precious and filled with wonder.

Return to the world when you are ready with a stretch and a smile! You have journeyed far, welcome home!

WILD FOOD

There is something powerful about the timelessness of foraging. Knowing that despite living in a world that our ancestors would be terrified of with its pace and noise and brightness, when we gather our food, medicine and beauty from the wild spaces we are taking part in an unbroken human ritual spanning tens of thousands of years, intimately connected to the Wheel of the Year. This in itself is profoundly healing.

The great woundedness of our time is our disconnection from the land. Foraging helps me to remake that connection. Increasingly, I gather very little when I forage but I try very hard to notice which green friends are present, to touch a leaf, to nibble here and there. It feels so important to take some wild food into my body as a prayer to life and to deepening relationship.

Jacqueline Durban

Foraging is a fabulous antidote to the hurriedness of modern life. It necessarily slows us down to the pace of nature. To our own natural pace. You have to be aware as you pick or you will prick your finger or sting yourself on a nettle or anger a wasp or bee. You have to shift your gaze to a deeper, slower way of seeing when you are gathering the more reticent of foods like mushrooms, learning again to see through the camouflage of the forest floor. You have to follow tracks and clues, get to know habitats, where to look and when. You must be alert to the unripe, the half-eaten, the maggoty, the poisonous lookalikes.

My passion for foraging and awareness of the ever-changing bounty of the wild edge spaces was cemented when, age ten, we were set a class project that was to take the whole school year: The Hedgerow Project. We were asked to seek out a local hedgerow and observe it over the course of the year. I thrilled at this invitation and spent the year noting the appearance of blackberries, sloes, rich red hawthorn berries and rose hips.
I was enchanted by the magic of jelly ear fungus and the black desolation of King Alfred's Cakes

emerging on rotting wood. The joy of the frothy white blossoms of spring, the tracks of fox and birds in frost and mud. The mystery of a gall appearing. Whilst most other kids compiled a short project in the last week when reminded about the assignment, I spent the whole year watching, taking photographs and samples, researching what I discovered in books. It set me up powerfully for my adult life – both as writer and witch. The awareness of what is there in the hedges year-round, what foods appear each year for a brief season, without us needing to do a thing was implanted in me. When I travelled through Australia, New Zealand and South-East Asia in my early twenties I relished tasting many things for the first time – magical-looking fruits like rambutan, mangosteen, custard apple and dragon fruit – but there were two things I missed as much as the people left at home: the hedgerows and my books.

In harvesting and gathering plants, we are connecting to both the plant and the world around us. In our foraging, we can connect to the wider world by mindfully leaving enough for other creatures, thanking the plants, and even help them to flourish by pruning back dead growth. The act of foraging itself has its own bounty of benefits, helping us foster mindfulness through immersion in nature, connection with the natural world and empowerment in seeking ones own sources of nourishment. There is a feeling of accomplishment from a meal that includes foods that you have foraged or grown yourself: a sense of connection with ancestral skills and knowledge, in our own small ways.

A recipe starts when you make the intention to create it.

The gathering of ingredients is in itself an important part of any foraged recipe.

I like to take a designated foraging basket or bag with me. I have a basket sitting by my door, ready to go, with a small bottle of some (old) fermented drink in it. This is to be offered to the plants and trees as I go by, especially to the ones I have gathered leaves from. This is only polite! Always ask the plant if it's happy for you to gather some of it. The answer is usually yes, but do be prepared for a no. You might not hear an exact word in your head, but receive a sense of yes or no. And offer something in return: your offering doesn't have to be a drink, it can be a hair from your head, a feather you've found, a pretty shell from your pocket…

I like to not be in a rush when going for a foraging walk, more like a dawdle, which we've been told is a negative thing (just sit and observe runners or walkers in public parks and you will see the idea of dawdling and observing what is around you has been forgotten). My ideal scenario is to do an intuition-led forage, where you let your intuition or inner-knowing guide you from one plant to the next. Firstly sink into your heart-space in whatever way you do this. Focus on your breath or putting hands on a tree, stand and truly observe something beautiful, say thank you and really feel it. Let your attention be caught by something. Sometimes it's an animal, bird or insect that points the way to the next flower or leaf. There can be such a gorgeous flow to this journey.

Fall back in love with the wild plants around you – your ancestors will love you for this. I'm saying 'back in love,' because there's an ancient knowing within you, a familiarity, that you can tap into.

Penny Allen

Our foods are part of who we are, and who our ancestors were, and tuning in to our cultural history through cooking can serve as a connection with the divine and ancestral lines. It can be a beautiful healing experience, taking the time to explore, play with and develop ancestral recipes, creating recipes that may be passed down to future generations, or simply creating using whatever treasures you have found on a certain day in the earth by your home.

It's more common now to buy herbs and tinctures than to forage and wildcraft them, but it is so beneficial to take notice of which plants are trying to attract your attention, and why, by showing up in your local area, even if you choose not to forage them. When I was studying homoeopathic nutrition, my teacher used to say that everything we need is growing right under our noses and I have found this to be true. During the pandemic self-heal (Prunella vulgaris) started popping up everywhere, and when I finally took notice of this amazing (but diminutive) plant I could see exactly why it was stepping forward for me: antiviral, anti-inflammatory, protective of the heart (physically and metaphorically). I tinctured it and it sustained me throughout that difficult time.

Jessica M. Starr

The thrill of a new season starting – cherry blossom, morels, carrageen, elderflowers, wild strawberries, meadowsweet, sloes, blackberries – is, for many of us, akin to the excitement of Christmas as a child, knowing that the window to gather these wild treasures is small. They must be sought out and transformed to preserve them.

In these times of plenty, most of these wild foods still cannot be bought in shops. They must be found. There are no guarantees. Your money is useless. Here you need sharp eyes, patience, local knowledge, seasonal and meteorological awareness and a good dose of serendipity. The harvest is so variable, reliant on the right mix of sunshine, showers and frost, at just the right time. It's you against the birds and other wild animals, as well as other foragers. Each discovery is a blessing. The finding of new places with rich pickings is a delight, and only shared with the closest of friends. A handful of browned fallen crab apples may seem insignificant to many, but they can make an apple sauce or chutney that brings nutrients and wild flavour to a meal or makes a precious gift for someone else. These little treasures have no value in a consumer culture, so are often ignored. But there is value here for those who seek to find it, putting small riches to good use. Seeing the value in wild things, being grateful for them, that's part of what it is to forage. In the grand tradition of witchcraft to see – and make – magic in places where others may not is the noblest of pursuits.

To forage is usually to gather what were once called 'need foods'. It should be done with the utmost respect for the plants and place, ensuring that you only gather what you need. It should always be done with some knowledge, of your own or from others, about when and how one should best forage so as to not damage the plant or creatures that may also have need of it.

Foraged foods are important in a lot of kitchen alchemy – as the kitchen extends beyond the walls and starts with where the ingredients have come from.

I love to connect with the seasons through foraging for what is abundant at the time and using it in anything I can! This enables conversation and appreciation for the land, the seasons, the cycles and connecting with the landscape and plants around us. Each plant can bring inspiration and creativity to the kitchen.

Milly Watson Brown

When we forage wild plants we take time out of our days to show up, prepared. We make the effort. We prunc and tend as we pick. We help spread spores and seeds. We remove litter. We re-connect with the wild Earth and our wild ancient selves. We recondition our palates to the wild bitter notes lacking in overly sweet modern foods. Eating as our ancestors did, as we evolved to eat. Gathering food together to cook and eat together. We nourish ourselves with micro-nutrients that modern growing methods and varieties are missing. We become reaccustomed to the wide variety and variation of shapes, colours and sizes that wild nature produces, rather than regulated conformity. And we remember, as we do, that humans too are allowed to be just as unique, varied and wonderful.

When we reawaken to the tastes of the wild, we reawaken to ourselves. Sun on our faces, wind in our hair, mud on our feet, thorns in our fingers, we are immersed in the magic generativity of this planet. We take only what we need, with respect, and give back. We begin to remember a different way of being.

Living by the cycles of the year, we begin to weave ourselves back into the natural world, relearning our kinship with the non-human, the basic magic of living interconnectedly that modern Western culture has forgotten. Rather than mere consumers, we learn to become active participants in the magic of life once again.

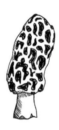
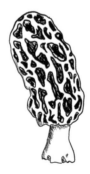

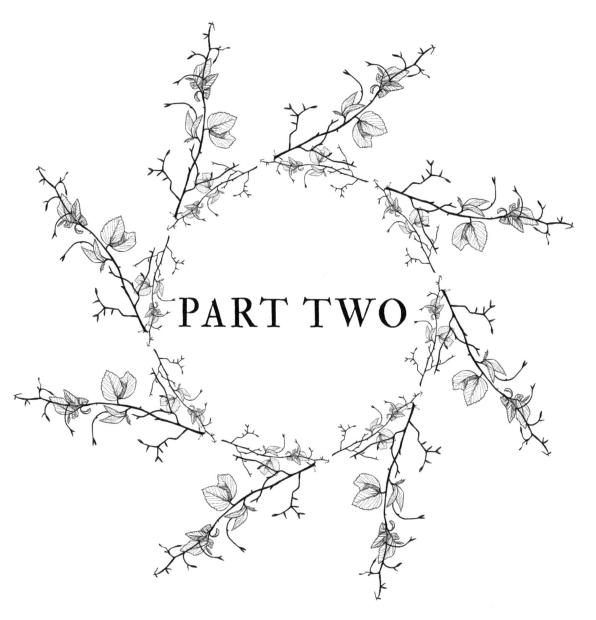

PART TWO

"Make for yourself a power spot
Bring you a spoon and a cooking pot
Bring air
Bring fire
Bring water
Bring earth
And you a new universe will birth…"

Shekhinah Mountainwater, from *The Goddess Celebrates* by Diane Stein

THE ART OF KITCHEN WITCHERY

This section shares recipes and practices for each season – you might choose to sprinkle them throughout your days, or have a couple of special afternoons set aside, perhaps one with friends/family/fellow kitchen witches and one alone, more contemplative. These add a good rhythm to our lives and years.

Our dearest hope is that this book contributes to you developing a more magical relationship with all aspects of preparing, cooking, eating and sharing food. That you are able to experience and savour the abundance of the natural world on your table. That through gathering, cooking and eating you develop a deeper connection to your inner wisdom, your intuition, as well as with your companions and the world. That you remember yourself as belonging to this Earth.

Often we pile our shoulders high with dreams, demands and expectations. Let them go, love. Allow yourself to drift and dream as you read the recipes and rituals in this section. Fully indulge your inner kitchen witches fantasies. Then set aside both space and time to make magic. Show up with that intention, with a recipe or spell, see what ingredients are abundant… and then leave space for magic. Magic shows up by itself, it cannot be forced. Remember in this moment you are no longer instigator but humble witness.

We have created a visual guide to the main practices of kitchen witchery, as we see it, to support you on your path. We have found that it is helpful to have a simple reminder of each of the practices to incorporate over the course of a season, in order to fully celebrate and embody all that the season has to offer. This list allows us to ensure that our practice is balanced, so that we don't get into the habit of thinking kitchen witchery means *I need to be cooking everything all of the time!*

☽ **Reflect:** take time alone in nature or your kitchen to think, write, meditate, bless, read…

☽ **Heal and cleanse:** yourself, those you love and your living space.

☽ **Ritual:** this might be spellcraft, lighting a candle or making sure you polish your sink each night.

☽ **Sow and gather:** what can you plant this season – practically and spiritually – in anticipation of times to come? What can you gather from hedge, forest, garden or shop?

☽ **Adorn:** decorate your kitchen and home seasonally with gathered natural beauty, homemade crafts or bought decorations.

☽ **Cook and craft:** what can you brew, make, create in your kitchen to nourish, preserve or delight?

☽ **Feast:** share food together, sing, dance, chat, laugh, drink and be merry… or create a special feast to celebrate one of your favourite foods.

PRACTICAL POINTS

ORGANISATION

This section is divided into four seasons, and each season progresses from early to late. Each part starts with an overview of the season, suggested kitchen table charms, crafts, and floral suggestions for wreaths and posies, as well as a meditation which you might want to do alone or share at a gathering. There then follow seasonal recipes including ingredients to forage for. Each season has cakes, cookies and treats, drinks, a soup, savoury dishes and a ferment. We have tried to group recipes that would go well together for the events mentioned and that celebrate the flavours and produce of each season. There are reflections on beloved seasonal celebrations and ingredients, as well as a spell, a simmer pot and a blessing for each season.

The recipes include many of our personal favourites. Some are historical recipes, some celebrate foraged or seasonal ingredients, some are magical looking or sounding – enchanting and delicious – and most have magical and/or medicinal properties. Many of the recipes are interlinked – either to be served together, or one using the by-products or left-overs of another to seed a new dish.

There is an introduction to each recipe from its contributor to contextualise it both historically and within their own food culture or personal life. After the recipe, we share the Kitchen Witch Magic: the healing and/or magical properties of the main ingredients, so that you can build your working knowledge as a kitchen witch and adapt and create your own magical recipes.

Some of these Kitchen Witch Magic insights are medically recognised, some are folk remedies, some are drawn from magical praxis, and some are drawn from superstition. The connections of ingredient can vary from practitioner, culture, and history. So, as always, take these notes as suggestions, not rules. We've drawn from some of the classic 'herbals' of Culpeper and Gerard and more modern Wiccan and Pagan texts as well sharing classical correspondences and interesting snippets of lore. Of the many contributors who have shared their recipes, some have included magical properties of ingredients, some have not. There are so many ways of treasuring food, so we love this variety, rather than a strict compendium or reams of listed correspondences (many useful and wonderful books do feature comprehensive lists of correspondences – if that is what you're seeking, our bibliography at the end of the book is full of ideas).

We also share the Celebrations that the recipe is suited to.

We have included accounts of some of our most memorable rituals and celebrations where many of these recipes were served and shared, in the hopes that they might inspire you to create your own special celebrations. Do note that some festivals have movable dates, such as Easter or Diwali. Seasons in the Southern Hemisphere are the reverse of those in the Northern, so, for example, Samhain is celebrated at the end of April in Australia. We have tried to deal with this as much as possible by talking about both seasons and months.

There is also a difference in tradition between different people and countries as to where the seasonal dividers lie, usually according to climate… for some in the Northern Hemisphere February is the first month of spring, for others it is March. For more on the history and customs associated with most of the seasonal festivals mentioned here, refer to the first book in the Kitchen Witch series, *Kitchen Witch: Food, Folklore & Fairy Tale*.

Whether you mark the festivals we describe here or not, we hope that the following section acts as a helpful guide to celebrating the seasons throughout the year. If you are able, seek out the local customs in your area like, apple and pumpkin picking in autumn (popular in both Europe and America) and summer BBQs on the beach of freshly caught seafood (popular in Britain, America and Australia).

The year as we have outlined it is one of memory, experience, joy and connections rather than a strict template or structure. Because day to day, that's how many of us live, finding special moments of unexpected sunny weather, quiet afternoons, gifts of vegetable gluts, a surprise guest dropping by, birthdays, baby showers, anniversary suppers…

Some of our recipes are made to feed two, others four or even ten. Some work better for large numbers and are great for taking to potlucks and celebrations, or hosting parties. Many of these recipes are also very handy if you like to batch cook in advance and freeze.

INGREDIENTS

Most of the recipes in this book need simple ingredients, which are easily accessible. We talk you through why each has been chosen, magically and nutritionally, so that you are empowered to exchange one thing for another to make your own magic.

Many of the seasonal and festival recipes we have included have ingredients that are native to Britain and Europe but also those that are available in North America, Australia and New Zealand, though they may well ripen at different times, or be more readily available in grocery stores than in the wild. The best advice is always to go outside in your local region and see what's happening. Part of the joy of foraging or observing your local wild spaces is tuning into the rhythm and seasons of your particular area. If you take regular visits into nature, you will find you can begin to connect to the plants there and predict the ripening of certain fruits and berries.

To cook is to create. And creating cannot be bound by finite rules! So, for all these recipes do not be afraid to add more spices, or swap fruits, vegetables and herbs for those that are available, affordable and bountiful. Some attempts will be a glorious success, some you will learn from!

Neither of us – or our contributors it seems! – are fans of following strict recipes, but we understand that this is necessary when trying a recipe for the first time, ensuring the intended texture and balance of flavour. Whilst we encourage creativity, bear in mind that most baked goods – there is an abundance of cakes, cookies and bread in the book, for which we make no apology! – do require precision and careful measurement of the main ingredients, but herbs, spices and other additions can often be interchanged, and we often offer several variations.

Bear in mind that if you are using dried herbs their flavour is stronger, so use half the quantity if replacing fresh herbs in a recipe.

Dietary Needs

Each of our bodies have different foods that heal or harm them. Each has different food memories of comfort and disgust. Each of us has foods that upset the balance of body or mind, that sicken not heal. Each of us has different foods we will and will not eat, because of cultural conditioning, health reasons or values. And these can change over the seasons of our lives.

We each have different relationships with our dietary needs and restrictions: for some we resent them and how they narrow our choices, (Sarah considers her lactose intolerance to be a terrible injustice, cream is awesome, for Lucy wheat has become a food which brings frustrating repercussions), for others dietary restrictions are freely chosen and add to our sense of self as well as our physical health. Many of us, especially in today's food culture, may have periods of eating one way, followed by another.

Our recipes here reflect these different dietary needs and allow for flexibility. Most can be adapted, exchanging one type of sweetener for another, plain flour for gluten-free, or dairy products for non-dairy alternatives.

Each recipe is marked at the beginning as to whether it is:

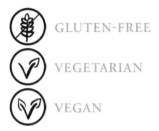

GLUTEN-FREE

VEGETARIAN

VEGAN

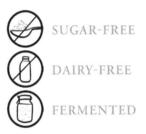

SUGAR-FREE

DAIRY-FREE

FERMENTED

Terminology

We are both based in the British Isles and so many of our recipes reflect this in terms of ingredients and cultural history. We have also drawn recipes from our international coven, so measurements, terminology and availability of ingredients might differ for you depending on where in the world you live, we have done our best to make these as accessible as possible to all our readers.

Weights and Measures

This book is written for an international audience – so we list measurements in three formats: metric, UK imperial measures and US measures. (The modern kitchen witch also has the magic of Google to find instantaneous ways to convert from one measurement to another!) We recommend that you choose one and stick with it for the duration of a recipe.

US friends please be aware, for reasons unknown to us, US pints are just under ½ a cup smaller than UK (imperial) pints (which are what we use in this book).

UK pint: 568ml (2½ cups)   US pint: 470ml (2 cups)

Sterilising Jars and Bottles

Sterilising jars and bottles is essential when it comes to preserving jam, chutney or sauces so that we aren't trapping any bacteria within. This extends their shelf life. In sterilised jars jams and chutneys can last many months – and even years – in a cool, dry, dark place.
There are a couple of ways you can do this.

How to sterilise jars in the oven

☾ Wash the jars and lids thoroughly and rinse clean. Do not dry with a towel.

☾ Place a sheet of baking paper on one of the shelves of your oven and place the jars, spaced apart, on the shelf.

☾ Heat your oven to 140°C / 275°F / Gas mark 1 and dry out the jars for 15–20 minutes.

How to sterilise jars by boiling

Like with baby bottles, you can boil your jars and bottles on the hob, useful if you just have a few jars or if you are using Kilner jars with the rubber orange seals. Again, wash your jars and the lids with hot soapy water and rinse.

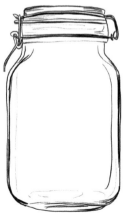

☾ Place the jars into the pan and fill with water just below the rim.

☾ Bring to the boil, and simmer for at least 10 minutes.

☾ After 10 minutes turn the heat off and leave the jars until you're ready to use them.

It best to use jars as soon as you can after sterilising.

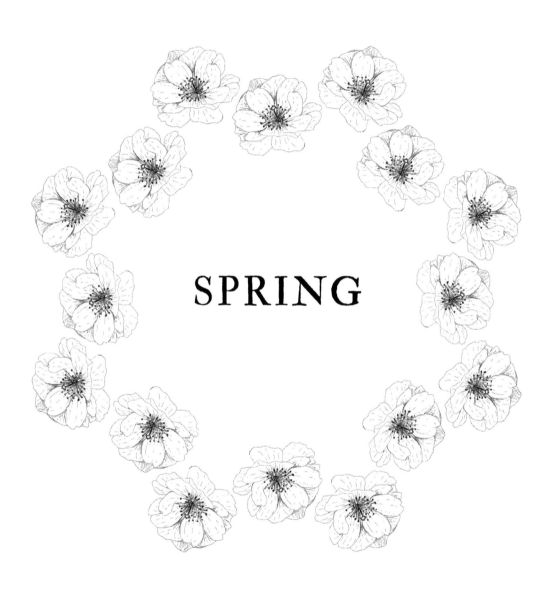

SPRING

Spring is the time to celebrate the rebirth of the year as new shoots spear their way through the ground and out into the springtime sun. Things are rising: the sap in the trees, new shoots through the earth, and the sun a little earlier each day. Tender leaves of nettles and wild garlic (ransoms) are at their best. You may be able to gather crisp leaves for gathered salads or the first flowers. Perhaps you look forward to an Easter feast with your loved ones with such treats as roast meat, eggs – chocolate or hens' – fruited breads and cakes.

A late afternoon in spring is the hour of long shadows and changing light: the best time to see the hidden glades where we may discover the bluebells have blossomed, wood anemones upturned to the sunlight that shines through fritillaries like fairy lanterns. Pale daffodils dance in spring breezes, and pussy willow catkins burst into tiny plumes. Woodlands and hedgerows begin to wake up.

All is fresh, crisp and green in the forest and the meadows. Leaves appear on the trees, and blossoms form bright white frills on trees and hedgerows, bringing a sense of hope and possibility for the coming season.

Some festivals and celebrations of spring include: Imbolc, St Brigid's Day, Sile's Day, St Patrick's Day, Spring Equinox, *O-hanami* (cherry blossom picnic), Passover, Easter and Ostara.

KITCHEN TABLE CHARMS

SPRING FLOWERS

Spring's floral beauty is best displayed as posies in jam jars and vases: primroses, daffodils of all shapes and sizes, branches of cherry, plum, apple and pear blossom (picked when in bud to bloom inside), flowering currant, bright green spurge *(Euphorbia)*, tulips in myriad colours, grape hyacinth…

☾ Display bright daffodils and catkin twigs in tall glasses. In Irish lore yellow is a colour of protection: daffodils, primroses, dandelions and gorse, the spring is full of them.

☾ Arrange posies of beautiful blues: forget-me-nots, muscari (grape hyacinth), bluebells (cultivated, not wild, which are illegal to pick in the British Isles) – blue is a colour of peace, protection, health and knowledge.

☾ String garlands *(lei)* of cherry blossoms to adorn your heads or necks, or the trees when celebrating *o-hanami* (cherry blossom picnic). The ruffled multi-petaled ones work best.

☾ And then there is the Brigid's cross, traditionally woven by householders on St Brigid's Day (1st February) from rushes, kept and displayed to protect the home for the coming year.

SEASONAL MEDITATION: SPRING

I describe a visualisation here, but do feel free to live out the actions described in this meditation! A morning dance in the sun is always a joyful thing and could be part of a simple and powerful ritual.

Close your eyes and relax as you settle and breathe.

We'll take a little time to visualise this amazing time in nature of expanding energy and warmth. Like the rising sun in the east, this is a new dawn and a new season, so together, in our mind's eye, we will watch the sun rise. See yourself stepping out of shadow, out of the dark winter, and the cold, and into the light of the morning sun.

Pause to bask in the morning sun.

This is a time of growth, of movement and blooming. So perhaps in the full light of the sun now, you connect to your primal spirit and move, dance, play in nature, and leap over fires! Listen deeply to rhythms and inspiration that arise. Feel the light of spring and summer dance into the air, dancing light around you.

Pause

Finally, allow yourself to unfurl like a flower bud: have a good stretch and reawaken! And welcome back to the room and to the day!

WREATHS, POSIES AND GARLANDS

Cultures around the world gather seasonal flowers and leaves with meaning and combine them – weaving their stems or stringing the flowers to adorn the heads of maidens coming of age, women getting married, the necks of honoured guests and sacred statues, tabletops for celebratory meals and doors for festivities. The term 'wreath' generally refers to a sturdy circular arrangement, often hung on doors or placed on graves as memorials. A garland is a long string of flowers or leaves and a posy is a small bunch of flowers. All three are beautiful ways to adorn your home with the bounty of the season: flowers, fruits and foliage. They are great for gathering and making together with friends or children and make beautiful, biodegradable seasonal decorations or gifts.

They can also be made from all sorts of other materials – crochet, knitting, fabric scraps, felt, paper and upcycled materials. Flags, bunting, paperchains… there are so many creative ways to mark festivities with colour and pizazz.

Basic Guidance for Wreath-making

Wreath-making for the kitchen witch is far more than just floristry. It is about working with the plants and seasons…witnessing, gathering, preparing, weaving and adorning your sacred space.

Base your colour palette on what is available – in autumn this is usually warm oranges, reds and golds, in winter this might be dark greens and reds, in spring blues and yellows, in summer whites, pinks and purples. You can find more about the symbolism of colour in the section on Candle Magic.

You may choose to purchase some elements to supplement what you are able to gather from your garden or the wild: artificial berries or flowers, tinsel, lights, decorative motifs, baubles, raffia or ribbons.

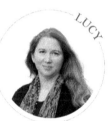

I love to decorate my door with a wreath most seasons – it's a beautiful celebration of what's growing and way to welcome guests to your door. I am not that handy with flower decoration, but wreaths I love. One Christmas a friend and I even had a business making them!

I have crocheted a garland for each season which I hang over the mantelpiece: spring flowers for springtime, sunflowers for summer, leaves and berries in browns, crimson and gold for autumn, and snowflakes for winter.

Gather your flowers, foliage and berries, ensuring the stems are at least 5cm long (2in) for ease of construction. Use scissors or secateurs so you do not damage the plants. Pick plants which have abundant leaves and foliage to spare and which are reasonably hardy – anything which drops its petals whilst you are picking it will be too delicate!

Ensure you have a variety of different textures, leaf and petal shapes and sizes. Pick not just with aesthetics in mind, but also the symbolic meaning and healing qualities of each plant. We are aiming in all aspects of the wreath to create balance and harmony.

Make or purchase a willow, wire or woven vine base, 30–40cm (10–15in) across. To make your own cut some lengths of willow or ivy stems, at least 80cm (30in) long, shape them into a circle and bind with string or florists' wire so that they create a solid base for your wreath.

Weave in the greenery first, and any longer stemmed flowers, ensure the ends of the stems are on the reverse of the wreath, being sure to keep a visual balance. Weave in one direction so that there is visual flow. Next add in shorter stemmed flowers, berries and any other decorations you are using, using thin florist's wire to attach.

In order to balance the decorations, bring to mind the pentagram – the five-pointed star within the circle. Ensure that your decorations are evenly distributed between all five points.

Attach each element of the wreath well, especially if it is to be worn or displayed outside, so that it stands up to wind and movement.

Depending on the purpose of your wreath, weave in healing intentions, prayers for protection, precious memories for grave wreaths or for door wreaths to visualise welcome to all who will call to your home.

A Wreath for Spring

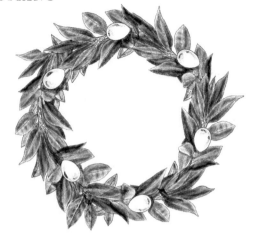

Spring wreaths can be woven from fluffy silver-grey pussy willow and dangling catkins, yellow forsythia, the furry buds of magnolia and the first crinkled leaves of beech. The cooler air this time of year helps wreaths last longer than an arrangement on your kitchen table would. To make an arrangement for inside make sure fresh leaves and flowers are in oasis or a bowl or vase.

EARLY SPRING

Gluten-Free Soda Bread

In Ireland soda bread is the traditional bread, raised with bicarbonate of soda rather than yeast. It is a simple bread that requires no kneading or rising. It can be ready in just over an hour. Served warm from the oven it is delicious thickly buttered with jam, cheese and chutney, peanut butter, hummus, or beside a bowl of soup. This is our everyday bread, and this gluten-free version was painstakingly developed by my husband after his diagnosis with coeliac disease, longing for good bread. It is a moist, nourishing loaf that keeps well for nearly a week, and toasts up deliciously.

Lucy

A note on buttermilk: Buttermilk can vary hugely from brand to brand – some being almost as thick as yogurt, others closer to milk consistency. It often separates in the carton so be sure to shake before using. If you cannot find it in your local shops read on for a recipe for making your own.

A note on oats: The oats you need here are the small crumbly oats which we call porridge oats in the UK and Ireland, used for making oatmeal/porridge. You do not want to use the sturdier rolled or jumbo oats here. Oats themselves are gluten-free, but those that are certified gluten-free (as required by those who are coeliac) are usually more expensive as they are grown, processed and packaged in a way that there is no possibility of cross-contamination from other gluten-containing cereals.

Makes one loaf

500g (18oz / 5 cups) porridge oats (gluten-free if required)

2 large eggs

450ml (16fl oz / 2 cups) buttermilk (or 420ml milk with two tablespoons of plain yogurt)

60ml (2fl oz / ¼ cup) flavourless oil (sunflower, canola or vegetable oil)

2 teaspoons honey or (brown) sugar (omit if sugar free)

2 teaspoons bicarbonate of soda (baking soda)

1 teaspoon fine salt

A handful of nuts/seeds – we love walnuts, pumpkin seeds, sunflower seeds, chia and sesame.

Regular rectangular loaf tin (1lb loaf tin)

Preheat oven to 180°C fan (190°C / 350°F / Gas mark 4).

Put one teaspoon of oil in a loaf tin and put it in the oven whilst it is pre-heating.

Remove a tablespoon of oats and set aside. Pour the remaining oats into a large mixing bowl. Sift in the bicarbonate of soda so that there are no lumps, add the sugar and salt and stir to combine. Add any nuts and seeds you want.

Mix all the wet ingredients – buttermilk, oil and eggs – together in a jug. Pour most of the contents of the jug into the bowl, reserving the last couple of tablespoons of liquid. Stir to combine. It will be a moist mix, much wetter than a yeasted bread dough. You want all the oats to be well-coated and sticking together, with no extra liquid floating around. Dependent on your oats and buttermilk you may need to add the last bit of liquid.

Remove the tin from the oven. Carefully spread the hot oil over the base and sides of the tin with a pastry brush or piece of kitchen paper. Sprinkle the tablespoon of dry oats you reserved to cover the base of the tin. Tip the bread mixture in and press it down gently to flatten it. You might choose to sprinkle with chia or sesame seeds on top.

Bake for 30 minutes at 180°C fan (190°C / 350°F / Gas mark 4), then turn the oven down to 150°C fan (160°C / 310°F / Gas Mark 2) for another 30 minutes. Take out of the oven and carefully loosen the edges with a palette knife. Turn out of tin onto a wire cooling tray. Carefully touch the bottom, if it feels damp, pop it back into the oven upside down out of its tin for 5 minutes to develop a crisp bottom crust.

For best slicing results leave it to cool for at least 10 minutes so that it doesn't crumble too much when you cut it.

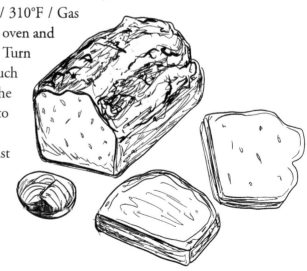

76

Kitchen Witch Magic:

Oats: for abundance, comfort and fortitude.
Buttermilk: the value of buttermilk can be seen in many folk tales of buttermilk being stolen by fairies, house spirits and witches. Rich and delicious, buttermilk is highly valued in many cultures and is connected to strength and prosperity.
Baking Soda/Powder and Yeast: raising energy and momentum

Celebrations:

Nothing comforts and fills the belly like bread. This soda bread would be a fabulous accompaniment for St Patrick's Day or Imbolc feasts, as well as perfect for bringing to group celebrations – housewarmings, New Year, fresh starts… According to Gaelic tradition to walk over a threshold of a home with bread means those who dwell within shall never go hungry: a fine gift indeed!

CULTURED BUTTERMILK

The watery liquid left over after the butter forms is called buttermilk. This can be cultured and used in baking and other cooking. A naturally fermented food, it is good for the gut biome. The bacterial cultures used for buttermilk are in the same family as those used in yogurt making.

In Ireland, buttermilk is a basic ingredient used in our daily bread – soda bread – as well as scones. It is also a core ingredient in American pancakes, some chocolate cakes and in fried chicken as it adds a tangy lightness to the batter, activating the baking soda. When used with meat it also serves to tenderise it. Cultured buttermilk also features heavily in ranch salad dressing, along with mayonnaise and chives, to create a tangy refreshing sauce.

Cultured buttermilk can be found in even the tiniest of rural corner shops in Ireland, whereas elsewhere in the world it can be quite tricky to track down. Which is why having a recipe here for it feels so important. You will need to source some buttermilk for your first batch. But after that you can carry on re-culturing indefinitely once you do it within a two-week timeframe.

If you have none to hand, and no time to make any, you can approximate cultured buttermilk by stirring a tablespoon of (unsweetened, preferably live) full-fat yogurt into each half pint of milk, it adds tang, thickness and culture, but does produce a heavier baked good. The other work around often suggested is adding a teaspoon of vinegar or lemon to your milk, but whilst this adds the needed acidity and thickens the milk a little, it doesn't aerate your baking in the way that cultured buttermilk will.

Lucy

3 tablespoons cultured buttermilk (bought or homemade)

425ml (¾ pint / 2 cups) dairy milk

1 clean, dry 1 pint bottle or jar with a tight fitting lid.

Pour the cultured buttermilk and milk(s) into your clean jar.

Screw on the lid tightly and shake vigorously. Place in a warm (but not hot) area out of direct sunlight (an airing cupboard is perfect) and leave it there for 12 to 24 hours, until thickened. Store in the fridge and use within two weeks.

A Bannock for Imbolc

 GLUTEN-FREE IF USING GLUTEN-FREE OATS

In Scotland's past bannocks were an essential part of everyday life, but also to any celebrations of the Quarter Days. Each festival had a bannock named for it, for example the *bonnach Brìde* for Imbolc (February 1st in the Northern Hemisphere).

On the eve of St Brìde's (Brigid's) Day it was customary for mothers to give out gifts of bannocks and butter to the girls who visited each house in the area with the *brideog*, the Brìde's doll. The making and the giving of the bannock was a ritual to ensure the prosperity and well-being of the household. A bannock might also be left out as an offering for St Brìde as she visited homes and farms to bless them.

Different parts of Scotland make different types of bannock, some more like soda bread, some with fruit and some more akin to shortbread. But essentially all bannocks are unleavened and can be cooked on a girdle (Scots for griddle/skillet) making it ideal sustenance on the go or in the fields.

I first made a bannock for an Imbolc celebration with friends in February 2020. I wanted to share a dish from my Scottish roots with my Irish friends. The occasion stands out as very special in my memory as it was the last time we met to share food together before the first Covid-19 lockdown.

The bannock I make is like a cakey oatcake, flavoured and embellished with delicious and healing herbs. You could change the herbs to suit the occasion or for any healing or magical properties you wish to induce.

Rosemary is ideal for Imbolc as it is an herb said to be sacred to Brigid and is usually still thriving in the garden in February. Rosemary increases circulation and is a stimulant, so it is ideal for the cold months. I also love to embellish my bannock with a scattering of dried lavender after baking. Lavender is relaxing both for the body and the mind and is said to help bring spiritual understanding to everyday life.

Leigh Millar

Serves 4–6

100g (3½oz / 1 cup) rolled oats

175g (6oz / 1 cup) oat flour (whizz rolled oats in a blender to make a fine flour consistency)

¼ teaspoon salt

6 tablespoons (75g / 3oz) unsalted butter, chilled (traditionally fat or dripping was used such as bacon or goose)

110ml (4fl oz / ½ cup) milk (plus one extra tablespoon for the caudle)

2 tablespoons chopped fresh rosemary (1 tablespoon dried)

1 teaspoon grated orange zest (optional)

3 tablespoons of sugar (and a little more for sprinkling)

1 egg yolk (for the caudle)

Grease a cast iron griddle (skillet) or, if using the oven, line a baking sheet and preheat oven to 190°C fan (200°C / 400°F / Gas mark 6).

Place the oats, flour, salt, sugar, rosemary and orange zest in a large bowl, mix together with a fork. Rub the cold butter into the flour mixture. Stir in the milk until a rough dough is formed.

Place the dough on a surface lightly dusted with oat flour. Knead until the dough is smoother but don't overwork.

Divide the dough in half and roll out each half into a circle about ½cm / ¼in thick.

Make the caudle – in small bowl mix the egg yolk with a tablespoon of milk. Then brush the mixture over the top of the bannock. Sprinkle with sugar.

Score each circle into 4 wedges.

Bake for about 20 minutes, until golden and crisp at the edges but soft in the middle. Or if using a griddle, cook over a medium heat on both sides until golden. Add more caudle if necessary.

Kitchen Witch Magic

Orange: bright and zingy, orange is often used to symbolise the sun or fire element.
Eggs: a symbol of new life with another sun symbol within – a sunny round yolk!

Celebrations

Imbolc (St Brigid's Day) celebrations of the sun, and any day that needs a little brightening.

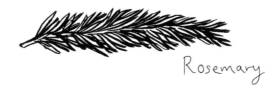

Rosemary

Tree Tapping

Penny Allen

Trees are energetic beings like ourselves, and as such are citizens of our community, whether we know it or not. I've experienced first-hand the generosity of the spirit of trees and the healing and happiness they can generate in us. By honouring and respecting them we can learn so much about ourselves.

Once a year comes the opportunity to drink the sap of trees, when the sap is rising, just as the leaf buds of the trees are forming and before they open into leaves. This is usually the two weeks after the Spring Equinox (around 21st March in the Northern Hemisphere) but different species come into bud at slightly different times, depending on their preferred temperature and light levels.

Many species of trees can be tapped, maple syrup being the most well-known. In parts of Europe you can buy birch sap in cartons from the supermarket. The three most common kinds of trees to tap are birch, maple and walnut.

Trees must be treated with respect. A considerate way to do this is to sit with the tree and ask it in your heart whether it would be happy to be tapped. You might get a feeling of a yes or a no. Don't be shy in doing this! Trees want us to ask things of them!

I have a special connection to sycamore, so it's no surprise that this is the tree I've had the greatest success with.

There are a couple of different ways to tap a tree but I find the easiest and least damaging way is just to cut the end off a small branch about 2cm in diameter, as if you're pruning. A small droplet of clear sap should form at the cut, indicating the sap is rising. If nothing forms, you're either too early or too late in the season. Pop a bottle over the end – tie this on with a piece of string so that it doesn't get dislodged and leave it to drip into the bottle overnight. Angling the tree branch so that the cut end is lower than the junction on the trunk can be helpful, as well as securing it down gently with a length of string.

I like to walk to the tree before breakfast and drink the sap in situ in deep gratitude to the tree and all of nature around her. I like to leave an offering, which is only polite. I usually bring some leftover fermented drink but this offering could be anything from a shell, stone, feather, hair from your head, pee, spit, bread scraps, ribbons. Sometimes, to adorn them, I make tree necklaces fashioned from wire, shells and feathers.

The sap itself tastes like crystal clear water with sweet overtones, each type of tree tasting slightly different. It is really refreshing, like an electrolyte drink: hydrating and balancing. It is lovely to share with family and friends. It revives and fortifies the body with natural sugars and minerals after the winter, and is deeply grounding and rooting to place. We have to trust nature's wisdom in the fact we can only drink the fresh sap for a couple of weeks in the year. I feel it wouldn't be beneficial to drink it year round. I guess with making a syrup from it to preserve it (as with maple syrup that we get in the shops which is boiled down) you're (hopefully) only going to consume it sparingly.

PICKLED MAGNOLIA

I only recently discovered that you can eat one of my favourite spring flowers: magnolia. One of the earliest flowering trees, the waxy white and pink tulip type flowers emerge on the wintery bare branches, setting Instagram alight with pictures of them blooming against powder blue spring skies. They have a flavour reminiscent of Japanese pickled ginger. Use the left-over vinegar for salad dressings. They can also be added to gin. Or made into a syrup for desserts and cakes.

Lucy

Petals of six magnolia flowers, washed and packed tightly into a sterilised glass jar

150ml (5fl oz / ¼ pint) rice wine vinegar

35g (1½oz) sugar

Pinch of salt

Bring the vinegar up to the boil to dissolve the sugar and salt, then pour over the petals right up to the top. Seal and keep in the fridge.

Kitchen Witch Magic

Magnolia: one of the first flowers to bloom in the chill air of spring. According to *The Complete Language of Flowers,* "some believe that a magic wand fashioned from the wood of the Chinese magnolia will bring the magician closer to working with the core magic and spirits of the ancient Earth."

Magnolia blooms contain two interesting compounds, magnolol and onochiol, which are anti-inflammatory, antimicrobial, and antioxidant and are also considered effective in reducing stress and anxiety and helping bring one to balance.

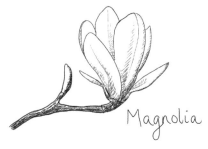

Magnolia

Celebrations

Magnolia blooming is always cause for celebration! Your blooms may appear early for Imbolc or later for Ostara, in which case they may be part of the festival feast. You may also use them for any occasion that calls for balanced thought, such as big decisions, an offering for forgiveness, or graduations.

A Celebration of Soup

Soup is a magical food in many ways that warms and nourishes both body and soul on grey days. It packs many vegetables and herbs and healing stock into each mouthful, sneaking vegetables past picky eaters. A smooth soup is easy to eat for the very young and very old, as well as the sick and recuperating. It is a fabulous way to make a feast out of bits and pieces, and a way to stretch ingredients to feed a crowd. It is a perfect dish to stash in your freezer. Soup makes a quick lunch, especially handy for those not eating wheat. Add a tin of beans or some leftover cooked grains to bulk it out. A grating of cheese, a drizzle of cream or olive oil to enrich it. It is no wonder pretty much every culture has a soup of sorts. A one pot wonder that can be bubbled over the fire, stirred occasionally, added to as needed.

We offer you a soup for every season…except high summer!

WATERCRESS SOUP

   CAN BE MADE VEGAN, DAIRY FREE

I grew up in Portsmouth, and Hampshire has a tradition of growing watercress – so much so as to have a 'watercress line' railway, in honour of the trains transporting watercress to the fresh produce markets of the UK during the boom in popularity in Victorian times. As a child I would ride on this train when it ran on special occasions. If we were lucky we were treated to my mum's watercress soup when we got home with plenty of bread.

Sarah

NB: Watercress can be foraged from fast flowing streams in many temperate climates. Be sure that you are not picking downstream from where sheep are grazing as the water may contain liver-flukes.

Watercress

Makes 4 generous servings

1 heaped tablespoon butter (or vegan alternative such as olive or sunflower oil)

400g (14oz / 3 cups) leeks, washed and chopped

700g (1½lb / 5 cups) potatoes, washed and chopped (peel if you like)

250g (9oz / 6 cups) watercress, washed and chopped

560ml (1 pint / 2½ cups) stock of your choice – enough to cover all the veg

4 tablespoons crème fraiche (or vegan alternative)

In a large pot, heat the butter and add the leeks, potatoes and watercress and stir them around so they are coated in butter. Gently soften for 15–20 minutes.

Add the stock and seasoning.

Simmer for a further 10 minutes, or until the vegetables are tender. Turn off the heat and use a wand blender to whizz the mixture into a velvety green soup. You can scoop batches into a traditional blender or do a rough mash with a potato masher if you don't have a magic wand! (Some people prefer a chunky soup – if so, you can skip this step entirely!)

Make sure the soup is piping hot (reheat a little if needed) and serve in warm bowls, stir in a swirl of crème fraiche to each bowl and garnish with a few fresh watercress leaves.

Kitchen Witch Magic

Any recipe passed on through friend or family holds a connection to ancestral magic.

Watercress: connected to the element of water making it cleansing, purifying and refreshing.

Leeks: the national emblem of Wales and powerful symbol of protection.

Potatoes: earthy grounding, soothing, calming.

Celebrations

Spring Equinox, Ostara, St Brigid's Day, any celebration of new growth or new ventures.

SPRING FORAGING

When we asked our coven of kitchen witches their favourite wild food to forage, by far the most commonly named was not mushrooms or berries but… nettles! Each had their own wisdom and trusted recipes.

The best foraged foods are those which grow in profusion and can be easily identified. My preference is for the new greens that come after winter's long reign – wild garlic, and the first of the new nettles. I like making nettle soup, but I also wilt them down with spinach, or mix them with feta in little pastries. They wake the blood up and nourish us with iron. Wild garlic, I feel, wakes the senses up, and is excellent in spells for invigoration and warding. It can also be made into the most beautiful bright-green pesto.

Alice Tarbuck

I think my favourite foraging is the gathering of nettles. They are simply divine and have many layers of gifts for us. Firstly, the gentle sting which tingles your fingertips whilst picking, increasing your circulation; followed by boiling the kettle and popping a couple of tops in to a mug to enjoy as a nourishing, cleansing tea; then chopping them and adding to your cooking – whether sautéed in a stir fry, steamed with your carrots, added to a soup or curry or blended into smoothies – nettles are so versatile and nutritious. They are rich in iron, vitamin C, calcium and protein to name a few. In my opinion they are the greatest, most versatile and abundant free food out there.

Milly Watson Brown

Packed with nutrients and medicinal constituents, these edible wild plants—often considered 'weeds'– are deeply nourishing. When you eat these wild herbs, the lines between food and medicine blur . . . and your food becomes your medicine. And that nourishment is not only physical! Harvesting wild greens reinforces your energetic connection to the land on which you dwell. I also consider our bodies and the plants to be sacred . . . and I find that the experience of harvesting and eating these gifts of the Earth nourishes body and soul.

Corinna Wood, corinnawood.com/blog/wild-edible-plants

A History of Nettles

Nettles have long been a staple in herbal medicine. Britain's **oldest recipe** (not written but discovered via archaeological study) is believed to be a nettle pudding, and dates back to the Mesolithic era – around 6,000 BCE! Ancient Egyptians are thought to have used them to treat joint pain, while Roman soldiers apparently rubbed nettle leaves on themselves for warmth (and perhaps to raise the inner fire for fighting). Their Latin name, *Urtica dioica,* is drawn from the Latin 'urere', which means to burn, and that burning sting of the plant means it is often connected to the element of fire and protective magic. The leaves can be dried and have been used in sachets by witches to ward off negative energies.

Nettle

Harvesting Nettles

The following recipes call for fresh nettle tops.

Look for the bright green growth, which will look different from the duller and darker green of the old leaves. Ideally only pick nettles growing above hip height (to avoid contamination by dogs) and don't pick in areas which might have been sprayed with pesticides or other fumes, like on the sides of roads. If you're hardcore then you can harvest the nettles without wearing gloves. If you grasp the tip quick enough then you usually don't get stung. But, full disclosure, I wear gloves when harvesting, though I do leave an offering to Mars as an alternative to the pain price of the sting.

Jessica M. Starr

NETTLE PESTO

   CAN BE MADE VEGAN, DAIRY FREE

Pesto can be made from many herbs – basil pesto is the recipe many think of, but when I'm in the mood for pesto I've also used mint, parsley, coriander; literally whatever green thing is in my fridge or garden (or red, I've used sun dried tomatoes too). Italians make a nettle pesto in springtime, they call it *pesto d'urtica*. This is my very basic pesto recipe for using springtime nettles, but if you find yourself with some wild garlic or some wilted coriander from the back of the fridge, feel free to use what you have. I love pesto on my pasta, but you can also add a dollop on top of such delights as cheese on toast, baked potatoes or scrambled eggs.

Sarah

Enough to cover pasta for 2

40g (1½oz / 1 cup) nettle tops

3–4 tablespoons of olive oil

70g (3oz / ½ cup) cashew nuts, lightly toasted

1 clove garlic

2 tablespoons Parmesan cheese (or vegan cheese)

Juice of half a lemon (for extra 'zing' and to preserve the vibrant green colour) (optional)

Just whizz this all up in a blender (if you don't have a blender you could also mush it up in a pestle and mortar but it will be a little coarser). Add a little more oil or lemon juice, or a small splash of water to get the consistency you like. If you have some leftover put it in a small bowl and cover with a thin layer of olive oil to prevent oxidisation before covering with a lid or cling film. Like this it will happily last a week or more in the fridge.

Kitchen Witch Magic

Nettles: rich in minerals and vitamins, nettles can be used to reduce inflammatory ailments. Nettles are full of nutrients, perfect for nourishing the body as we unfurl from winter and move into spring.
Cashew nuts: high in magnesium, nuts in general are a symbol of fertility and prosperity – useful for sympathetic magic.

Celebrations

Ostara, Beltane, celebrations of growing warmth and light. Or to invoke the energy of this warmth when it is lacking – such as in cold dark weather.

SUPER SPRINGY NETTLE SMOOTHIE

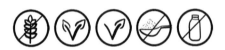

I love that time of the year when the nettles start to show vigorous, bright green, new growth. The daylight is noticeably longer now, spring has sprung! This usually coincides (there or thereabouts) with the Spring Equinox. The Equinox marks the beginning of the astrological new year, when the sun crosses into the sign of Aries. Aries is a fire sign, ruled by the vigorous and assertive god Mars. It is an excellent time of the year to turn words into action. That martial energy fortifies us and helps us to believe in ourselves, to own our power and strength.

When you freeze, cook, or blend nettle it destroys the little hairs which cause the sting. So you don't have to worry that this recipe will be painful. It's actually really tasty and nutritious.

Jessica M. Starr

Serves 1

A handful (ouch!) of freshly harvested and rinsed nettle tops

A frozen banana (fresh is also fine, but frozen is creamier and keeps it colder)

Half an avocado (optional)

A tablespoon of nut butter, any type

1 cup of milk (dairy/soy/whatever you prefer)

1 cup of water with a scoop of vanilla protein powder (or another sweet ingredient like a couple of dates, or a teaspoon of maple syrup)

Add all the ingredients to a high-speed blender and blend for 30–60 seconds. The mixture will be bright green, thick and creamy. It's that simple. Even children love these smoothies.

Kitchen Witch Magic

Nettle: iron-rich, fortifying, for protection and courage.
Banana: for potassium and sweetness, energy and resilience.
Avocado: for good fats and creamy texture, protective.
Vanilla: soothing and balancing.
Nut butter: satiating and soothing.
Milk: soothing and a good balancer for the Martial energy of the nettle.

Other uses for nettles:

+ In oil…use for salad dressings and to make aioli.
+ With potatoes and kale in soup.
+ A steaming pot of nettle tea.

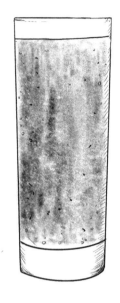

COLCANNON WITH WILD GREENS

   CAN BE MADE VEGAN

The first reference to colcannon is thought to be a 1735 diary entry of Welsh traveller William Bulkeley, who had the dish on Halloween night in Dublin: "Dined at Cos. Wm. Parry, and also supped there upon a shoulder of mutton roasted and what they call there Coel Callen, which is cabbage boiled, potatoes and parsnips, all this mixed together". Like bannocks, it is a treat that was often eaten on all festivals days from Imbolc to Yule, along with the fortune telling customs popular on these special days – for colcannon in particular, a coin and other items were cooked inside, and whatever charm you found in your potatoes predicted your future. Interpretations varied by area, but a coin usually means wealth in the coming year, and a ring signifies marriage.

Colcannon itself has many variations but is essentially mashed potatoes with cabbage and/or other vegetables mixed in. I like it when the weather is cold, or I don't want to cook anything complex. For a simple winter evening meal I put sausages in the oven while I boil the potatoes and veg in the same pan, drain and mash together and dish up with some gravy. In Ireland it is traditionally served with a boiled ham (bacon), which is delicious glazed in the English style in the oven for ten minutes slathered with English mustard and honey until it has a bubbly sweet crust.

The colcannon I cook most often during the winter is with cabbage, or leeks if we have some in the garden. But come spring, the possibilities of using foraged wild greens appear. This is my perfect recipe because it really doesn't matter how much of anything you use. Lots of people over? Use more potatoes! Lots of greens to use up? Add more! You'll still end up with colcannon at the end, so I'll tentatively say, it's foolproof!

Sarah (and Lucy!)

(Feeds two hungry people)

4 large potatoes, chopped and peeled

Handful of wild greens of your choice and/or green cabbage or kale, shredded

50g (2oz / ½ stick) butter (or dairy free alternative)

75ml (3fl oz / ⅓ cup) mixture of cream and milk (or dairy free alternative)

2 spring onions (scallions) or bunch of chives (optional)

Steam or boil the potatoes for about 20 minutes, for the final 10 minutes add your greens, which may be cabbage, kale, chopped sprouts, or wild greens like nettles, wild garlic, sorrel, dandelion leaves or yarrow (wild greens need less cooking time than cabbage and kale, so drop it down to 5 minutes simmer time if using these). Drain, and return to the pan. Add the butter and milk and mash. Season well with salt and pepper. Serve with an extra knob of butter melting on it, and perhaps a sprinkling of spring onions (scallions) or chives. (Adding in charms is optional!)

Kitchen Witch Magic

Cabbage: the leaves have been used in British folk medicine to reduce soreness and swelling, especially of nursing breasts. Chewing cabbage was traditionally prescribed for headache, cold and flu. The cabbage patch is also connected to birth and babies: in Victorian England babies were said to arrive from cabbage patches (to avoid referring to any unseemly bodily or biological functions). So cabbages can support starting new projects of any kind.

Potatoes: have also been used in British folk medicine to reduce soreness, especially of rheumatism. They are also grounding, as all root veggies are, which can make them comforting and soothing.

Celebrations

Often enjoyed at Celtic festivals such as St Brigid's Day, St Patrick's Day or Samhain. Using seasonal green veg can connect the dish to a seasonal or regional celebration. Also useful as a simple fortifying meal before starting a new project or journey.

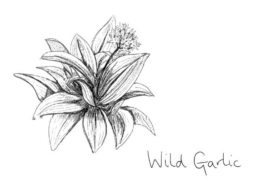

Wild Garlic

Simmer Pots

Sarah Napoli

Herbs from the garden in a cauldron black, bubbling and boiling as their earthy scents fill the space. Slices of citrus fruits cleanse and purify the air as the ingredients brewing here become one, combined together for a magical purpose. Simmer pots, at their start, were used as a liquid pot-pourri to freshen the home and create a warm inviting space. To the modern witch a simmer pot is not only seen as a scent enhancer but as an opportunity. An opportunity to create magic and intention in our own kitchen, the place, I believe, is the true heart of the home.

In my home everything happens in the kitchen. It is where I enjoy meals with my family, it is where I craft my herbal remedies, and it is where I have ended many days with a cup of soothing lavender tea as the sun goes down. In my personal practice, simmer pots have become a staple for setting magical intentions. Taking ingredients, whether that's herbs, fruits, or water that has basked in the energy of the sun or moon, to create magic in the mundane. As a new mom, time can more often than not be crunched. Learning to adjust my craft and find ways I could create magic, while still being present as much as I need to be for my little one, has taken a while. Simmer pots allow me to utilize a variety of ingredients and set intentions, all while doing the laundry and making a bottle. They are a fantastic way to combine, create and craft a little bit of magic in the chaos that is everyday life.

In this book I share some of my most cherished brews celebrating the natural cycles of the Earth in the form of seasonal changes. Spring, summer, autumn, and winter all hold their own beauty and correspondences. The same can be said for the phases of the moon or the days of the week. My hope for these potions is that you will be able to honor these cycles, work with them personally, and be able to craft these spells in your own kitchen.

But the magic doesn't stop at the spell, the steam, and the scent. There is much more to be utilized from a brew such as the ones you will find here. As a folk and nature witch, repurposing and reusing is a large part of my personal magical practice. Once your pot has simmered and that magic has been infused, that water becomes a sacred tool. It can be used to consecrate altar spaces or tools with your set intention. It can be used as a door and floor wash for the home, spreading that intention even further into the space. Fruits can be composted for garden preparations or dried out for later spell work. You may even choose to soak up this intention by adding a splash to a ritual bath.

Get creative and begin to see these ingredients through a different lens that allows you to get the most out of your simmer pot. When crafting these brews you may choose to dedicate a specific vessel such as a cast iron cauldron or saucepan that is used only for these magical purposes. Get to know the plant allies you are working with, not only for magical purposes but medicinal as well, to make sure the ingredients you are using may be safe for a ritual bath soak or any furry friends you may have close by. I do hope you find inspiration in these recipes and draw from them to craft and create your very own simmer pot potions.

Spring Cleaning Simmer Pot

Spring is all about rebirth, new beginnings and planting seeds. Letting go of the old to make room for the new. The blooming flora is colourful and bright and the floral aroma makes the home feel just as refreshing and crisp as the first day of spring. This pot is intended for clearing old energy and creating a fresh space for new things to thrive and grow. This brew is also a perfect one for repurposing as a wash for your doors and windows, for any physical cleaning and cleansing you may be incorporating into this ritual. Always check your ingredients to make sure they are safe should your furry friends come in contact with them.

Sarah Napoli

For this brew you will need:

Water charged under a New Moon.

Lavender for calming energy.

Tiger lilies for uplifting the mood.

Calendula for joy and happiness.

Rosemary for good health and vitality.

Lemongrass for balance and love.

Cinnamon for success and abundance.

Combine your ingredients. Stir clockwise and say:

> *Spring is now here to cleanse and to clean,*
> *Making room for these intentions to flow through to me.*

Allow to simmer as long as desired and add water as needed.

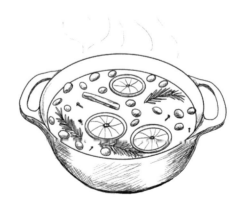

LATE SPRING

KITCHEN TABLE CHARMS

Coloured eggs

Easter's association with eggs runs back into the ancient past. Eggs are a symbol of rebirth and fertility, hope and expectancy, as well as precious protein after a long winter.

Start with white hard-boiled eggs, cooled to room temperature. We'll soak the eggs in a simple dye bath.

The dye bath: Put half a red cabbage and water enough to cover it in a large pot, bring to a boil and simmer for 40 minutes. Take off the heat and remove the cabbage (which can be used for soup later or composted). Let the liquid cool at room temperature. Stir in 2 tablespoons of white vinegar. Then soak your eggs in this mixture for at least half an hour; for darker colours, let them soak overnight.

Remove the eggs from the staining liquid and place them on paper towels to dry completely.

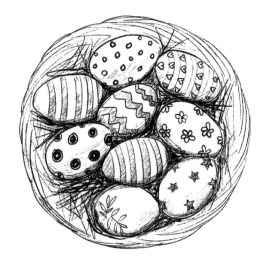

Edible Flowers

Edible flowers have come back into vogue, adorning salads and desserts in upmarket restaurants, for a pop of colour and finesse. They are chosen for aesthetics and occasionally flavour. The kitchen witch harnesses many facets of the flower, including also its traditional symbolic uses (both from folklore and the more recent Victorian language of flowers), the symbolism of its colour, number of petals, the goddesses they are associated with, as well as their medicinal and nutritional benefits.

We love to cook with flowers and will be sharing some of these different properties alongside many recipes in this section.

Great ways to use edible flowers include: cocktails, mocktails and teas, salads, decorating cakes, candies, chocolates and cookies.

Not all flowers are edible, but lots are. (Always check if you're unsure, foxglove and nightshade are two to avoid for starters!) Here's a non-exhaustive list of wild and cultivated edible spring and early summer flowers that work well with the recipes in this book:

borage

chamomile

cherry blossom

clover flowers and leaves

cornflower (petals)

daisy (lawn)

dandelion petals

dianthus (commonly known as "pinks")

elderflower

flowering currant

forget-me-not

jasmine

lavender

lilac

marigold petals (calendula)

meadowsweet

nasturtium

primrose

pansy

rose (petals)

rosemary flowers

strawberry flowers

sweet (scented) geranium

Sweet William

thyme

viola

violet

Be sure to pick away from dog pee and pesticide/herbicide sprays, wash or at least tap the flowers to get rid of any creepy crawlies. Generally with flowers just use the petals as the stems and sepals can be tough and bitter tasting, sometimes inedible.

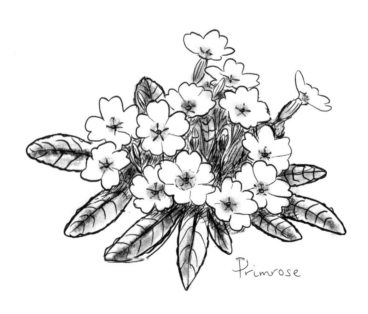

Primrose

Spring Flower Shortbreads

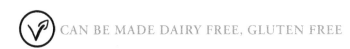 CAN BE MADE DAIRY FREE, GLUTEN FREE

If you loved flower pressing as a child, or still do (I don't think most of us grow out of it!) then this is an edible equivalent…but much faster! The whole process is a joy for a last-minute special-looking treat to go with a cup of herbal tea for an impromptu tea party in the spring sunshine or as a loving handmade gift. You start off with a wonderful excuse to head into your garden or the nearest woods to pick some spring flowers as the super simple dough is resting. Then you get to press the flowers into the tops of the shortbreads. Herb sprigs that work on sweet biscuits include: sweet cicely, sweet woodruff, lemon balm, mint and lemon thyme.

You can also chop up fresh or dried lavender flowers or dried rose petals and add to the dough if you would like some extra floral flavour.

Be sure to take a pretty picture before you pop them in the oven. Bake the shortbreads for ten minutes and the flowers come out looking like they've been pressed for a month. Magic!

These are beautiful served with a sprinkle of sugar on top, or exquisite with strawberries and cream, or a bowl of freshly made lemon or passion fruit curd drizzled on when cooked.

From beginning to end they take maximum twenty minutes to make! The only way you can go badly wrong is to overcook them. Watch them like a hawk after the first five minutes – under done is better than over done with these, they go bitter if they get too dark. You are looking for a pale golden colour.

You can use gluten-free flour, but it gives a slightly gritty texture.

You can replace butter with non-dairy alternative and leave out the egg (you may need to replace it with a couple of teaspoons of water). The dough will be a little crumblier and not so easy to re-roll.

Lucy

Makes about 30

300g (10½oz / 2¾ cups) plain flour

200g (7oz / 2 sticks) cold butter

100g (3½oz / ½ cup) caster sugar
(plus 2 tablespoons for serving)

1 large egg

Preheat the oven to 170°C fan (180°C / 350°F / Gas mark 4).

Rub the butter with the sugar by hand or using a food processor until it resembles fine breadcrumbs. Add the flour and mix to combine. Then add the egg or a little water. (Add the rose petals or lavender if using at this point). If using your hands bring it together into a ball, kneading it slightly until it is in one big lump. It will automatically come together in the food processor. Be careful not to overwork it as the gluten will become activated and the shortbreads will be chewy not crumbly.

Wrap and chill for 30 minutes in the fridge. Pick and prepare the flowers, knocking off any little bugs and removing stems.

Violet

Lightly flour a clean surface. Roll the dough out to ½cm / ¼in thick with a rolling pin. Cut out using a medium (5cm / 2in diameter) round or heart shaped cookie cutter, or a floured glass and place onto a non-stick baking sheet. Using a wet finger press the flowers onto each shortbread.

Bake for 8–10 minutes, watching carefully. Remove from the oven when pale golden. Leave on baking sheet for 5 minutes then transfer to a cooling rack. Sprinkle with a couple of teaspoons of caster sugar.

Savoury Version

Whilst wild garlic and chive flowers are very pretty, I wouldn't advise adding them to sweet cookies, unless you want a strange flavour clash!

To make a savoury version, omit the sugar, and add the same amount of cheese as butter (grated mature cheddar, parmesan or Gruyere, or a mixture of these) and a grinding of black pepper. Before baking, top with borage, wild garlic or chive flowers, or sprigs of dill, fennel, thyme, parsley, sage or rosemary or perhaps some baby beech, nettle or hawthorn leaves… maybe adding some chopped herbs or wild greens into the dough for extra flavour.

These are delicious served with a whipped cream cheese thinned with a tablespoon of cream with a big bunch of chopped herbs and/or wild greens mixed through.

Kitchen Witch Magic

The Victorians developed a complex language of flowers, a way of communicating feelings to suitors and friends in a culture that did not allow an open expression of passion of any sort. The following are some meanings according to the traditional Victorian language of flowers if you wish to send a message with your baking! You will find that some align with traditional magical correspondences and others are quite different.

Primrose: youth
Rose: love
Purple (dog) violet: faithfulness
Yellow violet: rural happiness
Rosemary flowers: remembrance
Thyme flowers: activity
Pansies: thought
Elderflower: zealousness
Strawberry flowers: esteem and love
Nasturtium: patriotism
Borage: bluntness or courage
Chamomile: energy in adversity

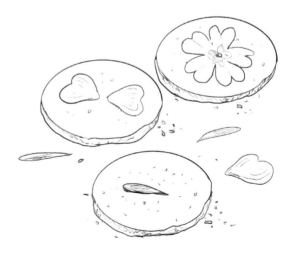

Celebrations

Turn up at any home or gathering with freshly made biscuits and you will be very popular! Use floral messages if you wish such as yellow violet for a cottage housewarming, chamomile for one facing a challenge, or primroses for a baby shower.

Gathering – Cherry Blossom Picnic

For me the beauty of spring is encapsulated in the appearance of the cherry blossom. Delicate, ethereal, a visible sign of new life and hope: the ghostly promise of glowing fruit yet to come. The white or pink flowers standing in their vulnerability on bare branches, braving the chill air, before the leaves have unfurled from their buds. They fall like snow, blessing the ground with their pale petals.

In the days before we had children, my husband and I lived in Japan for a year, just like my father before me. My father had always described the extraordinarily romantic nature of the people of Japan – especially where cherry blossom was concerned. Every spring throughout my childhood he would sing me their ode to the cherry blossom.

We fell in love with the cherry blossom, with Japan, and with each other – I proposed to my husband during our time in Kyoto, completing a sacred circle, as I myself was conceived there on my parent's honeymoon!

In Japan cherry blossom is used as a metaphor for the fleeting beauty and vulnerability of life. In late March and early April, in parks, gardens and along riverbanks around Kyoto, you would find *o-hanami* – cherry blossom picnics – in full swing. Many in traditional kimonos. All out to celebrate the season's snow-petal beauty.

After telling my children stories of *o-hanami* when they were little, it was decided that we must have our own. And so we have every year since. Some years under leaden grey skies, wrapped in coats and hats against the chill spring air, others in short sleeves under sunshine and a powder blue sky.

Finally peak blossom arrives on the cherry tree in our garden and we can wait no longer. We prepare butterfly cakes filled with cherry blossom jam (recipes to follow!) and spring flower tea. The tea was a revelation the first time we made it. It lifts the spirits in the gathering… and the drinking. We gather what is abundant in the garden: wild primroses, violets, some early wild strawberry flowers and leaves, scented geranium leaves (but you could use lemon balm or lemon verbena instead) and, of course, cherry blossom, and add them to boiling water in our floral teapot. Drinking it steeps us in the delicate taste of spring.

We lay out the blanket and pile the tiered floral cake plate with cucumber sandwiches, pink and white marshmallows, butterfly cakes, macarons and spring flower biscuits and adorn it with cherry blossoms. We fill our cups with steaming spring flower tea and feast together, the snowy blossoms bobbing above our heads.

Lucy

CHERRY BLOSSOM JAM

One year, for our cherry blossom picnic, I decided to make cherry blossom jam from the petals. We used it, along with whipped cream, to make our cupcakes into butterfly cakes, a traditional English tea-time delicacy.

If you only have white blossom to hand you may want to add a drop of pink food colour, a hibiscus flower or a raspberry to add a beautiful pink colour to your jam.

Cherry blossoms have a very delicate scent and flavour, reminiscent of almonds. They need minimal cooking, as it affects the flavour.

Petals have no pectin, which is the substance that thickens jams, so you either need to use jam sugar that has pectin added or you can add an extra teaspoon of lemon juice. In the summer this recipe can be used with rose petals to make rose petal jam.

Lucy

Makes 1 jar

225g (8oz / 1 cup) jam sugar OR caster sugar with 1 teaspoon lemon juice (see above)

1 cup of fresh petals shaken free of bugs, stripped from stamens, leaves and stems

170ml (6fl oz / ¾ cup) water

A couple of drops of pink-red food colouring / 1 raspberry / 1 dried hibiscus flower (optional)

If you have time, steep the petals in the water for 10 minutes to help the flavour develop. Add the sugar and stir over a medium heat until it thickens. Stir through colouring if using. Pour from the pan into a serving bowl or sterilized jar and allow to cool.

BUTTERFLY CAKES

This recipe was a mainstay of English children's birthday parties and summer fêtes of the 1970s, '80s and '90s. The fanciest of little cakes, offshoots of what are known as fairy cakes, were as indulgent as it got before the arrival of the larger American cupcakes with their massive indulgent swirls of buttercream.

The butterfly wing effect is created by cutting a circle from the top of the fairy cakes (leaving a small ring of cake around the rim). The removed circle is carefully cut in half to make the wings. The hole is filled with buttercream or whipped cream (which tends to have a blob of jam, curd or fresh fruit hidden underneath. The wings are then stuck on top. There is something rather magical about them for children and adults. Choose some fairy cake cases in a pretty colour or pattern (these are smaller than muffin cases).

I make these gluten-free as standard, if you want them nut-free and gluten-free just use standard gluten-free flour in place of the nuts, they will not be quite so cakey and moist. If gluten is not an issue you can replace the ground almonds with plain flour.

Lucy

Makes 9

For the cakes

100g (3½oz / ½ cup) caster sugar

50g (2oz / 2 tablespoons) butter

1½ teaspoon baking powder

25g (1oz / 5 teaspoons / ¼ cup) rice flour

25g (1oz / 5 teaspoons / ¼ cup) cornflour (cornstarch)

70g (3oz / ⅔ cup) ground almonds (almond meal/almond flour)

1 large egg

120ml (4fl oz / ½ cup) full fat milk

1 teaspoon vanilla extract

Filling

A third of a jar of jam or curd

250ml (9fl oz / 1¼ cups) cream, whipped

Preheat oven to 170°C fan (180°C / 350°F / Gas mark 4).

Fill a standard cupcake or muffin tin with pretty paper cases.

Using an electric hand whisk or food processor, blend the butter with the dry ingredients until it looks like breadcrumbs. Add the egg, milk and vanilla.

This is a runny cake batter, do not fear…it works! Spoon it into the cupcake cases so that they are two-thirds full.

Bake for 15 minutes, checking after 10. They will be risen, rounded golden domes. Stick a toothpick or skewer into the centre to test. No wet cake mix should come out.

Take out of the tins and cool on a wire tray for at least half an hour. These need to be completely cool to the touch before cutting the tops off and filling with cream otherwise the cakes will crumble and the cream will melt.

Put a teaspoon of jam into each hole and top with a tablespoon of whipped cream. Then place two 'wings' on, cut ends sticking into the cream, cooked sides facings inwards (see illustration). Dredge with sifted icing sugar.

FERMENTATION

Penny Allen

Fermentation is a subject as old as time itself. We as humans have learnt to harness the power of microbes to help us create beneficial foods and drinks (or some might say it's the other way round!) Fermentation is one of the witchiest things you can do: put herbs and other ingredients into a pot and let it bubble away!

The rhythmic, cyclical nature of fermentation connects you in a whole new way to the world around you. You create and support a mini microcosm when you ferment. It's like being a microbe farmer: you create a mini farm on your kitchen counter!

I always say there is nothing like doing something over and over to become intuitively connected to the process. Through observation and curation you become in tune with how your ferments develop: you become part of the process, part of the symbiosis. Through lived experience you learn from the smallest subtlest signs. Nuances in temperature, humidity, light levels, atmospheric pollution, energy levels, all these have a noticeable effect on fermentation.

We are highly sensitive beings that don't even realise most of our superpowers. Fermentation is one 'way in' to learning about fine tuning them. Observation is key in fermentation. Using all five senses and then learning to use your sixth sense, your intuition, makes for powerful and deeply healing ferments.

DANDELION LEMONADE

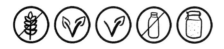

This lemonade is a fermented foraged fizzy drink with cleansing properties: it is a true celebration of spring.

It's so exciting when all the new plants begin to appear each spring. Where I live, in Ireland, this could be as early as the end of January. Dandelions can often be found throughout the winter in sheltered spots, but I love to make this recipe with the new growth each spring. I use dandelion leaves and flowers, as well as whatever wild plants are plentiful including: cleavers, young thistle leaves and young dock leaves.

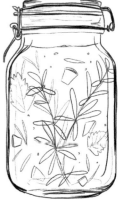

The quantities going into this drink are not necessarily medicinal ones, but I like to think that the sum of its parts is greater than that. We will never fully understand the synergy and interplay between plants and what happens when you ferment them together.

Be sure to wash any fruit to remove traces of wax or pesticide.

**1 x 1.5 litre (2½ pint / 1.5 quart) clip top glass (Kilner) jar and
1x 1 litre (1¾ pint / 1 quart) sterilised glass bottle**

20g (1oz) fresh cleavers

10g (½oz) fresh dandelion leaves and flowers

1 apple chopped small

250ml (9fl oz / 1 cup) fresh citrus juice
– I use 2 lemons and 2 oranges

½ lemon sliced

250ml (9fl oz / 1 cup) water kefir, kombucha or ginger bug (see p144)

75g (3oz / ⅓ cup) caster sugar

250ml (9fl oz / 1 cup) boiling water

700ml (1¼ pints / 3 cups) water

In a jug add the sugar to the boiling water and stir to mix till dissolved. Add the cold water to this and pour into the jar. Place the cleavers and dandelions into the jar and add the chopped apple, citrus juice, sliced half lemon and the water kefir/kombucha. Give it a good stir with your favourite wooden spoon or wand! Close the lid tightly and place it on a countertop at room temperature to ferment for two days. Sit this on a plate just in case of any leakages.

You should see bubbles of carbon dioxide forming, and the colour of the herbs will fade.

The best way to decide if it is ready is to taste it. It should be fizzy with a lovely balance between sweet, sour and bitter. When it is to your liking, strain the liquid through a sieve, composting the herbs. The apple pieces make delicious sour fizzy bites or you can whizz them into a smoothie or add to porridge.

Bottle into a 1 litre sterilised airtight bottle. Keep in the fridge.

Because this is fermentation, everyone's environment will impact the process with different temperatures and humidity.

Penny Allen

Cleavers

Kitchen Witch Magic

In English folk magic, dandelion clocks are often thought of as a tool for divination or used as something to be wished upon.

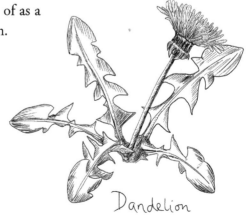

Dandelion

Rising Ritual: Spring and The Kitchen Witch Star Path

Using our seven-pointed star as guide, this ritual journey can be done as a group, on your own, or a combination of both. It may take an hour or be a journey over a weekend. This is a ritual specifically for spring and just one example of infinite ways to use the 7-pointed star path as guide…

Timing: for spring rituals morning is a great time to practice your magic.

1. Sow and gather – Select a pot or tub that will adorn a space in your kitchen, perhaps windowsill or light space. Select a seed – this in itself can be a mindful journey – perhaps take a walk to the great oaks in your nearby park and look for an acorn. Or take yourself out to lunch at a garden centre with happy memories and buy a cheery looking packet, or gather your fellow kitchen witches to swap seeds.

2. Adorn – Choose where this seed pot will rest in your kitchen and make the space sacred – this can be as simple as a wipe down with a cloth and some scented water, or you may create an altar or centrepiece with branches, leaves, seeds, items of use and beauty. The area you decorate can be as small or as large as you wish, from a windowsill to your whole kitchen.

3. Cook and craft – Take your time to brew a cup of tea/coffee and make a snack or sweet treat.

4. Feast – on your tea and food! You can do this alone or as a group activity.

5. Reflect – take time in quiet reflection or with your journal – *How do you wish to grow this season?* You can write down ideas, draw or make a vision board, or simply roll the question around in your mind.

6. Heal and cleanse – finish your little feast and wash your hands. With this simple act also think of washing away anything that may hinder your growth – as we prepare to use our hands for our simple seed planting ritual.

7. Ritual – Now it is time to plant your seed and water it as you speak aloud all you wish to grow this spring. Finish the ritual by placing the pot in its new home.

Seasons Blessings

Whatever your religious or spiritual beliefs, blessings are an ancient practice found in all cultures of sharing good intentions, positive thoughts and well wishes. When we speak or even think them before we eat or drink, be it together or alone, it adds an element of conscious awareness to our consumption, a moment of pause. All cultures share a word and a moment when folks gather to eat and drink together, a way of bringing the group together – Cheers! *Salud! Sláinte! Santé!* To your health! *Kampai! Itadakimasu! Bon appetit! L'chaim!* Enjoy! Welcome!

If you want something a little more elaborate for a special celebration we will share one at the end of each section.

May we be nourished and blessed.
May the abundance of this table overflow in our lives.
May this time together be held forever in our hearts.
"Bless the food before us, the people beside us, and the love between us."

Anon

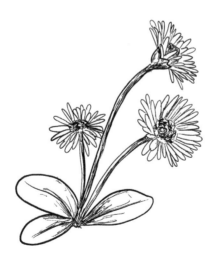

101

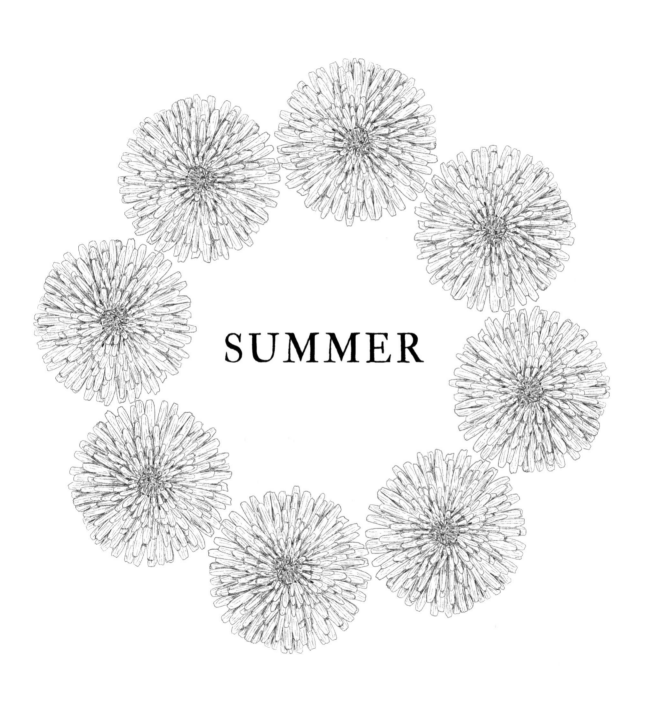

SUMMER

This is the season to pack up a picnic and wander over grass and meadow, the kitchen hearth moves outside with the fire of barbecues and zinging energy of games and laughter. We play amongst the scents of strawberries, lavender, and sun-ripened tomatoes and celebrate Midsummer, the longest days and shortest nights. Walk as slowly as you can to bask in warm sunbeams and marvel at hedgerow blooms, roses, sweetbriar, and blossoming honeysuckle, because before you know it, we'll move into late summer, fields ripening into soft gold under bright sun and warm breezes, harvest time begins…

Celebrations for summer include May Day/Bealtaine/Beltane, Summer Solstice/Midsummer's Day, Blooms Day, St John's Day…and a hundred opportunities for picnics, barbecues, outdoor parties, sports events, summer fêtes…

KITCHEN TABLE CHARMS

Roses, and lots of them! Arrange them with lavender, lemon thyme and geraniums for scent and colour to whisk you into midsummer's dream. And place in big vases, or picnic under them so that they may watch over solstice celebrations and feasting as symbols of love.

Perhaps display a jar of honey on your table or kitchen altar, in honour of all things sweet and abundant, and also the Mead Moon (one of many medieval European names for the summer full moons). Bees are a symbol of good luck, of course they are best left well alone in their hives – but if a bee lands on you or flies into your house it is considered an extra blessing for the season!

Summer Wreaths

The scents of summer make wreath-making intoxicating. Most summer wreaths are made of delicate flowers which have a brief lifespan – fresh summer wreaths are no good for doors as they will start to wilt after a couple of hours without water – you need to use artificial flowers for this. They are, however, beautiful for anointing heads at rituals and ceremonies, or displaying on tables for weddings or parties. For table decorations use florists' oasis or soaked moss or a vase of water to keep them hydrated. Keep cool for as long as possible, and mist with a water spray to refresh.

Fabulous summer flowers to work with include: roses (be sure they aren't a variety that drop their petals too easily and remove thorns for head garlands), lavender, rosemary, sweet pea, cosmos, baby's breath, montbretia, jasmine, hydrangea, heather, vetch and daisies of all sorts.

Kitchen Witch Magic

Lavender: soothing and calming, and suitable for all cleansing spells. The name lavender is drawn from Latin: *lavare* meaning 'to wash" (lavender was commonly used to scent laundry, clothing and baths in ancient Rome; and we fully encourage continuing this practice!)

SEASONAL MEDITATION: SUMMER

Close your eyes and relax as we settle and breathe.

In our mind's eye we walk along the hedges of a peaceful country village, past a little collection of cottages, with kitchen gardens and cottage gardens. Roses climb over doorways and wisteria cascades over walls and windows. It is a lazy sunny afternoon, you can hear a gentle hum of bees and can see butterflies dancing in flight through greenery, and the chirp of birdsong and flap of wings. Breathe in the scents of lavender, rose, sweet pea and honeysuckle. The multisensory song of summer is here, resplendent in the bright light of the sunbeams. Listen. Breathe. And smile.

Everything is blooming, and you feel joyful as you arrive at a little thatched cottage with tables outside, each with a colourful parasol and comfortable wicker chairs with cushions. You sit down and a kindly old lady appears. She brings you a cool icy glass. Little blue borage flowers – deep blue and star-shaped – top the glass and the drink is cool and refreshing. Then she brings you a bowl of juicy berries. She says with a smile, "We picked them just this morning." Raspberries and strawberries, cherries and redcurrants: juicy, bright, and shining still warm from the sun, topped with whipped cream and golden honey, and a sprinkle of vibrant green mint leaves.

You don't recall ever having a fresher or finer meal, simple as it is – as though summer could be served in a bowl. You savour every sun-warmed mouthful with total bliss.

In time you stand and offer to pay. The lady wraps her small soft hands around yours.

"No payment today," she says, kindly, but firmly. "This is the day of sacred pause, this is the day of gathering all the good things of nature –fruits, herbs and honey." She tells you that this very morning she and her community met in a great circle of stones, where people have for generations gathered to watch the sun rise. Tonight, they will light bonfires on the hills, and burn herbs to bless their animals, homes and farms. Today is the day for sharing the simplest and most powerful of magic – love, light and generosity. She asks you simply to pass on the light to any you may see on this special day. And to take pause and reflect on all that is abundant and what are you grateful for. The old lady smiles once more and invites you to stay as long as you wish in the garden. Peaceful, happy and so grateful for simple summer magic.

Pause, and return to the world when you are ready with a stretch and a smile!

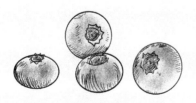 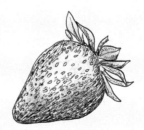

EARLY SUMMER

Elderflower Cordial

This, to me, is the taste of summer. Elderflowers are harvested from the hedgerows and made into sweet syrup each June. The cordial is served in most restaurants, cafés and homes in our area, either added to sparkling wine and cocktails, or served with still or sparkling water as a refreshing non-alcoholic drink. It is best in its first six months, it tends to go a darker colour and is less freshly floral as the winter draws in. In recent years commercial elderflower flavoured drinks have become available – the cheapest are artificially flavoured, the more expensive are just that, for something so cheap to make yourself from flowers and sugar in large quantities and bottled for the year ahead.

Try to gather the flowerheads away from busy roadsides on a dry sunny day for maximum pollen and flavour. Be sure to leave plenty of flowerheads to develop into elderberries for later in the year – for both humans and wildlife.

The citric acid can be bought from most pharmacies very cheaply. This white powder is used in commercial confectionery for its sourness and preservative powers, it is beloved of foragers for elderflower cordial and drug dealers apparently to cut their wares with, so many pharmacists can be unwilling to stock it or sell large amounts. It is not essential for the recipe, but extends its shelf life beyond a few weeks, and means you do not need to store unopened bottles in the fridge. If not using it add the juice of an extra lemon for extra tartness and keep refrigerated.

Lucy

Makes 2 litres (3½ pints / 2 quarts)

20 elderflower heads

2 lemons

1.2 litres (2 pints / 5 cups) water

1.8kg (4lb / 8 cups) sugar

60g (2½oz / 4 tablespoons) citric acid

Sterilised glass bottles

Shake the flowerheads to get rid of any creepy crawlies and remove any leaves. Dissolve the sugar in the water over a low heat. Shave the peel off the lemons in large strips using a vegetable peeler, then slice the lemons into circles. Put both peel and fruit into a large non-metallic bowl. Add the flowers and pour over the syrup. Cover with a cloth and leave overnight to infuse.

Remove the flowers and fruit (this is a sticky job!) and stir in the citric acid.

Strain into sterilised bottles through a muslin-lined funnel in order to remove any remaining petals, dirt or bugs. Seal and store in a cool, dark place. Serve diluted to taste. Store open bottles in a fridge. It is also lovely poured over summer fruits or lemon drizzle cake (see below).

Kitchen Witch Magic

Elder is one of the most magical plants in the hedge and kitchen witch's repertoire and was historically known as 'the poor person's medicine chest'. With anti-inflammatory and decongestive properties, it is used to treat colds and flu, asthma and hay-fever – which is on the rise as spring turns into summer. Elderflowers were commonly used to reduce heat in the body – so it is a beautiful and refreshing summer drink on many levels.

Sugar for sweetness and an energy boost. Sometimes used in spells of love to 'sweeten' someone up.

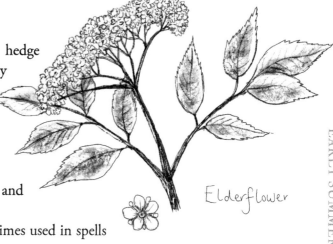

Elderflower

ELDERFLOWER AND LEMON DRIZZLE SQUARES

 CAN BE MADE GLUTEN-FREE

A bright zingy cake for spring and summer. These squares are fabulously quick to make, so perfect for unexpected guests or last-minute bake sale contributions. They're also great in packed lunches as there's no chocolate, cream or icing to melt. If you don't have any elderflower cordial to hand just increase the lemon juice and sugar that you top it with.

Lucy

For the cake

200g (7oz / 2 sticks) soft butter

180g (6oz / ¾ cup) caster sugar

200g (7oz / 1¾ cup) flour
(for gluten-free use 120g ground almonds, 50g rice flour, 30g cornflour/cornstarch)

4 large eggs

2½ teaspoons baking powder

Grated zest of two lemons

For the topping

Juice of 1 lemon

1–2 tablespoons caster sugar

2 tablespoons elderflower cordial syrup
(or 1 extra lemon)

Rectangular baking tray 30cm x 15cm (12in x 6in)
Preheat oven to 170°C fan (180°C / 350°F / Gas mark 4.)

Cream the butter and sugar together until light and fluffy, either with a wooden spoon or with an electric whisk/food processor/free standing mixer.

Add in the flour, eggs and baking powder and the finely grated zest of one lemon. Mix well to incorporate. Bake at 170°C for 30 minutes, checking with a skewer.

Combine the lemon juice, elderflower cordial and the zest of the second lemon.

When still hot from the oven poke several times with a toothpick, sprinkle with the sugar and drizzle the lemon-elderflower mixture over the surface evenly.

When cool decorate by scattering over yellow flower petals – dandelion, primrose or calendula – as well as individual elderflowers (no stems).

Kitchen Witch Magic

Yellow/orange flowers (like dandelion, primrose or calendula): good luck and positive energy, summer, sunshine, friendship and joy.

White flowers (like elderflowers): protection and peacefulness.

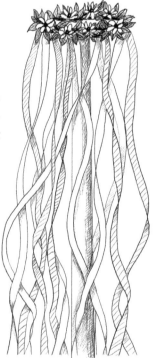

GATHERING – MAYPOLE

As a child at a small village school in England, despite its Church of England status, the seasons were marked in a semi-pagan way. Besides Christmas and Easter we celebrated Harvest Festival, Bonfire Night, and May Day. For our physical education classes for several weeks each year, we would get out the white-painted telegraph pole, hung with bright coloured ribbons, uncover the hole in the ground and slot it in. Then the traditional country dance music would be played and we would dance the ancient dances around the maypole in the sunshine, in a tradition that dates back hundreds of years, perhaps even to Roman times, and celebrates the returning fertility of the land.

When I had children in Ireland, this was one of the traditions I desperately wanted to pass on. I went online and ordered myself a maypole! My husband queried if we needed to spend quite that much on a long pole of wood which would be used once a year. So we got creative and made our own – repurposing the rusted metal poles from an old trampoline safety net to make the maypole, topping them with an old metal Christmas tree stand with a wreath of fresh flowers around the top and tied with ribbons. We invited over friends with similar aged children, I Googled the dance steps to refresh my memory and created a playlist on Spotify – a very modern approach to an ancient ritual which has become a much-loved tradition for another generation.

Lucy

May Wine

May Wine (known as Maibowle) is a favourite for May Day, especially in Germany. Like wassail (a festive warm ale and apple drink) in England, the contents can vary greatly, and it's the social elements that make it a ritual. Alcoholic versions use a sweet white wine (Hock, Gewurztraminer, Riesling or Liebfraumilch are all popular choices) or a honey mead (see recipe p174) as the base. This is then steeped with the leaves of sweet woodruff *(Galium odoratum)* – a delicate faintly aniseed flavoured herb, which is covered in white flowers at this time of year.

The sweet woodruff is usually picked fresh and then briefly dehydrated in a cool oven to release its delicate grassy aroma, before adding to the wine. The wine is left to steep for several days in the fridge, before straining. Strawberries are added to the glasses when serving. It can be served as it is, or topped up with sparkling wine or water for a celebratory feel. Other uses for sweet woodruff flowers would be for headdresses and altar flowers, as their sweet scent was thought to protect against malevolent spirits and bad luck.

Sweet Woodruff

Beltane Chicken

One of my favourite food-related rituals is the ritual suppers that my family have on the Sabbats. Among the favourites is Beltane chicken, which is roasted stuffed with a whole orange, to represent the sun. We serve it with saffron rice, some more sunshine-imagery, and it is always wildly greeted at table – and then we toast to the spring, and the coming year. It's a lovely family ritual, of candlelight and shared food.

Another thing I love is the first food cooked outdoors of the year – some of which is always offered to the Good Folk, to make sure they're included in the bounty. I like easy foods – pancakes cook well over an open fire, and sausages – and skirly, a Scottish stuffing, made with oats and sage, which is good with just about anything!

Alice Tarbuck

Kitchen Witch Magic

All meats are connected to abundance and good luck as feasting on meat was once, for many, a rare and special treat, often saved for particular occasions or festivals. Animals have been used in sacrifices and rituals by many religions, an uncomfortable but true statement (and obviously it is largely inappropriate and illegal now). They have a history in magical and spiritual practice. But whether you wish to use them in your cooking is a personal choice.

Chicken: in ancient Rome chickens were sacrificed to the gods and as the chicken is sacred in some parts of Asia and Africa, it is still sacrificed in Voodoo and Santeria rituals. Some cultures also still use chicken bones in divination, or the outlines created when chickens peck at grain. Chicken soup has long been associated with health and healing and the meat can also be used in food for good luck, fertility and prosperity.

Nettle Seeds

Jacqueline Durban

My favourite food to forage is nettle seeds. They are the most wonderful medicine for our ragged hearts as we continue to journey through all that we're facing in the world at this time. The seeds strengthen our skin and hair, support our kidneys, and strengthen our adrenal system. I have turned to them many times when under stress and found them a great comfort. Also, I love the danger of collecting nettles without wearing gloves; I don't recommend it, but I feel that the odd sting or two is a fair exchange.

The first time that I collected them I had no idea what I was doing and stung my hands so badly that I couldn't use them for two days. I was in a situation at the time that left me feeling powerless and losing the full use of my hands caused me to spend several days reflecting on the folktale of "The Handless Maiden", which is all about the wielding of power. Medicine comes to us on so many different levels.

Nettle seeds are incredibly versatile. They can be nibbled fresh from the plant and added to almost anything once dried. I like to make nettle seed oatcakes with them. They are delicious!

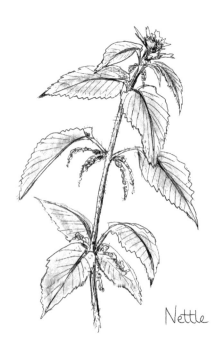

Nettle

Lilac and Nettle Seed Oatcakes

I can definitely taste a hint of lilac bitterness in these oatcakes, which I really like. I find them delicious on their own but they're lovely with butter or some cheese and/or chutney.

You can also make these without using lilac flowers, if you can't source any. They are lovely just with the nettle seeds. These oatcakes are not only tasty but also support us in times of stress.

Jacqueline Durban

140g (5oz / 1½ cups) porridge oats

140g (5oz / ¾ cup) oatmeal/bran

2 tablespoons plain flour – spelt is nice, use oat flour if keeping them gluten-free

A sprinkle of black pepper

½ teaspoon salt

2 tablespoons nettle seeds

2 tablespoons lilac flowers (fresh or dried)

A handful of mixed seeds (linseed, sunflower, pumpkin…)

75ml (3fl oz / ⅓ cup) oil (olive, sunflower, canola…)

Hot water

Preheat oven to 170°C fan (180°C / 350°F / Gas Mark 4)

Put all the dry ingredients in a bowl, mix and make a well in the centre. Working quickly, pour in the oil and enough hot water to make a firm, but not too sticky, dough. You will get used to how much if you make these a few times. If it gets too sticky you can add in a few more oats.

Rest the dough for 5 minutes and then roll out to around 5mm thick. Then cut out your oatcakes. I don't have a cutter so I use a glass jar. Or you can make the dough into balls and then flatten them for a rougher shape.

Put your oatcakes on a baking sheet and bake for 20 minutes. Turn them over and bake for another 10–15 minutes. Take out of the oven and remove from the baking sheet onto a wire rack to cool.

Kitchen Witch Magic

Nettle seeds: strengthen our adrenal system, which is often ragged from the pressurised and busy lives that many of us lead.

Lilac: can help us to negotiate the space between our domesticated and wild selves. Like a bird, she has hollow bones and can help us to hold our challenges more lightly. She is an important remedy for the back, especially for lack of flexibility in the spine but her healing essence is also of value at times when we need more flexibility in our interactions with the world, when we have become somehow locked into a situation or attitude, or when we need to 'grow a backbone' in some way. She is a bringer of both physical and emotional flexibility.

Lilac

Summer Picnics

Summer is a time of picnics: blanket spread out on the grass, under the shade of a tree in the afternoon sunshine, an array of tasty treats, a jug of homemade cloudy lemonade or perhaps an intoxicating glass of Pimms, floating with cucumber, fruits and borage flowers. And then there are the realities of nature to contend with – ants and wasps, thistles and prickles, pigeons, crows and seagulls, sticky fingers with nowhere to wash them and sand in your sandwiches. But regardless of these realities, the fantasy of picnics continues to lure us and food always tastes better outside in the warm, fresh air.

There are two sorts of picnics. The functional picnic to fill bellies, full of juice cartons, melted chocolate bars, squashed bags of crisps and sandwiches. And then there is the other. The carefully planned and cooked-for outdoor gathering, a lunch of salads shared on a rug, or an afternoon tea with steaming hot tea and tiered plates with a mouth-watering array of tiny sandwiches and dainty sweet treats – cakes, cookies, macarons, madeleines which taste of magic and memory. Many of the recipes in this book – fairy sandwiches, butterfly cakes, spring flower shortbreads, elderflower cordial and squares, butterfly pea or dandelion lemonade and tisanes – can be combined to make a magical afternoon tea.

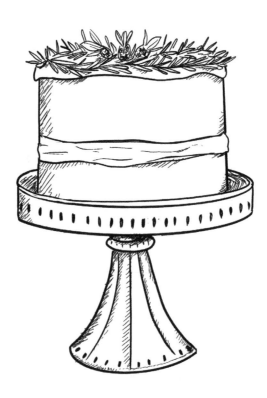

Butterfly Pea Lemonade

This drink is pure magic. The flowers are first brewed as a tea. Homemade lemonade is added. Do this in front of your guests for a **wow**, as the acid of the lemon juice instantly turns the tea from bright blue to purple.

Butterfly peas look like a sweet pea and a blue flag iris had a baby together. Their scientific name is rather fabulously *Clitoria ternatea* because of its visual similarity to the female anatomy (see image). A member of the pea family native to South East Asia they are easy enough to grow and can also be bought dried from herbalists, health food shops and specialist tea shops.

For a superlative magical brew, serve it with edible flower ice cubes, edible glitter or some borage flowers.

Lucy

Butterfly Pea

3 teaspoons butterfly pea flowers (fresh or dried)

700ml (1¼ pints / 3 cups) water

Juice of 2 lemons

Juice of 1 orange

Sugar syrup made from 110g (4oz / ½ cup) caster sugar and 150ml (5fl oz / ¾ cup) water

Ice cubes

Pour the boiling water over the flowers. Leave to steep for five minutes. Strain the tea and leave it in the fridge to cool. Add 1 teaspoon of edible glitter if using.

Meanwhile make a sugar syrup by dissolving the sugar and water over a medium heat. Leave this to cool in the fridge.

Add the juices to the sugar syrup and stir.

To serve fill the glass half full with the pea tea, fill to 75% full with the lemonade. Stir and add ice cubes.

Kitchen Witch Magic

Butterfly pea flowers: high in antioxidants with anti-inflammatory properties, they also stabilise the blood sugar and lift the mood. Also… a blue and purple drink, what is more magical than that?

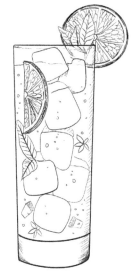

Fairy Sandwiches

I used to love fairies, and most especially the Flower Fairy books of Cicely Mary Barker. I would dress up as a fairy and hide at the bottom of my grandparents' woodland garden in the hope that I might catch a glimpse of these magical creatures.

After one such adventure I remember asking my mother: *What do fairies eat?* Why, fairy sandwiches and flower tea, was her swift response, which she probably lived to regret. For soon I was demanding fairy sandwiches for birthday parties and afternoon teas on the lawn! I have no idea if she got the recipe from somewhere or created them from her own imagination.

Made from bought sliced white bread (sliced pan as we call it, according to Irish custom) thickly buttered and sprinkled with multi-coloured hundreds and thousands. The soft, savoury bread, rich salty butter and crunchy sweetness of the sugar sprinkles was magic itself.

Lucy

Coloured sugar sprinkles/hundreds and thousands

Sliced white bread

Soft butter (I prefer salted)

Spread the bread thickly with butter and sprinkle generously with sugar sprinkles. Cut the crusts off – neither fairies nor children like them! Then cut into quarter squares, the slice each square into a triangle half. Adorn with edible flowers and petals.

Kitchen Witch Magic

Sugar, butter and white bread: here are some rather demonised items in the eyes of the diet industry – but their lightness and sweetness have always made them a favourite of the fae, and they may well bring a sense of magical indulgence and joy to your day as well.

Celebrations

Perfect for celebrations when fairies are thought to cross boundaries and roam the land such as Litha, Summer Solstice/Midsummer's Day, Lammas and Lughnasadh, as well as sunny garden parties and lazy picnics – if at all possible, young children should be present, dancing in their finest floral dresses, flower crowns and fairy wings!

Summer Solstice Celebration

I put on a purple dress and place a crown of flowers on my hair. I collect my small children and we make our way out into the cloud-dark rain to go to my sister-in-law's house for a Solstice fairy tea party with the cousins.

The table is laden with fairy lights and jewels and teacups are arrayed at each place. We eat miniature biscuits with homemade hedgerow jelly, lemon cupcakes with raspberry mascarpone frosting, and tiny brownie brownies as we drink ginger peach tea. Afterwards, we pool our resources and make fairy terrariums, bright green moss layered in glass jars with imitation butterflies, bird's eggs, and other small trinkets and treasures arrayed around the edges.

After dinner, we gather for our simple family Summer Solstice ritual. I originally planned to circle outside during sunset, mystical trails of incense drifting in the humid air as we created a flower mandala together. But it is overcast and drizzling. The little kids suggest a footbath ritual instead, and so we circle our chairs between the kitchen and living room, filling tubs of hot water and passing ritual salts, oils, and dried flowers around to one another. I decide to step outside briefly into the light spattering of raindrops and pick one Queen Anne's Lace blossom for each person as well as a handful of rose petals. The flowers are completely prone, weighed down with rain. As I look at the flowers, I see the wild, spontaneous, unconstrained wonder within them and some words of blessing trail through my mind,

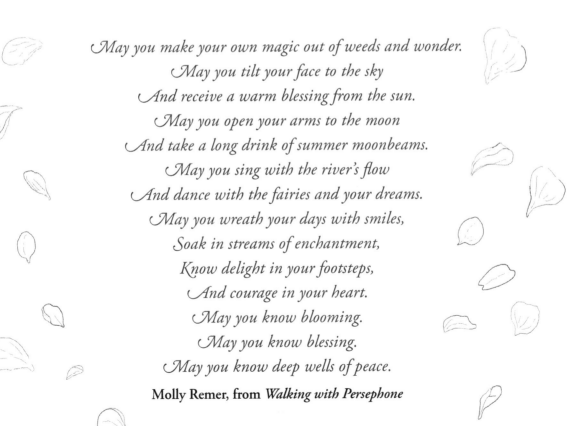

May you make your own magic out of weeds and wonder.
May you tilt your face to the sky
And receive a warm blessing from the sun.
May you open your arms to the moon
And take a long drink of summer moonbeams.
May you sing with the river's flow
And dance with the fairies and your dreams.
May you wreath your days with smiles,
Soak in streams of enchantment,
Know delight in your footsteps,
And courage in your heart.
May you know blooming.
May you know blessing.
May you know deep wells of peace.

Molly Remer, from *Walking with Persephone*

Midsummer Roses

I make no secret of my passion for roses. Not the tight-lipped imported ones, but the big blowsy, highly scented old-fashioned English ones that have graced the gardens of cottages and castles for centuries, which drop their petals in disdain as you try to pick them to adorn your table. The sort of roses that climb walls, whose stems bend and bow rather than stand to attention. There is nothing more sensual, exotic and heavenly for me, than the scent of roses: they are my favourite flowers. Roses have traditionally been connected with the divine feminine (probably because of their visual connection to a beautiful vulva). Long associated with fertility and sexuality and the goddess in many forms – Mary, Venus, Isis – they reconnect us with the sacred feminine through the body and our sensuality.

I have filled our garden with roses – light and dark pink, yellow, white…and even a rather odd lavender coloured one! But I don't celebrate them just for their visual beauty, or even their scent…but for their flavour too.

Lucy

Rose

Rosewater

An ancient anointing scent from the Middle East often used for blessing, rosewater can be used to wash hands or bless a forehead at the beginning of a ritual. It has been used in sweet and savoury recipes in English cookery since medieval times and Persian cooking for centuries before that.

It can be bought in supermarkets, delicatessens and Middle Eastern stores, but you can also make it yourself… in fact the chances are you probably did, as a magic potion as a child in your plastic bucket, stirred with the nearest magic wand (stick) you could lay your hands on… and then probably forgot about it in the sun until it was a slimy stinky brew.

To make your own rosewater, fill a jar with pure water (boiled, bottled spring or distilled water) and a handful of scented (unsprayed) rose petals, ideally picked on a sunny dry day. Cover and leave on a sunny windowsill for a day to infuse.

For a faster version, add a handful of scented (unsprayed) rose petals to a saucepan and top with enough water to just cover (no more or you'll dilute the flavour). Bring the water to a simmer over a medium-low heat and cover. Simmer for about 20 minutes or until petals have lost their colour. Then drain through muslin into a sterilised bottle, seal tightly and keep in a cool dark place.

The same methods work for other scented flower waters such as lavender or orange blossom.

Wild Rose

CRYSTALLISED ROSE PETALS

Crystallised flowers are beautiful for decorating cakes and desserts. Crystallising preserves the petals' colour and flavour to a degree, making them crisp, sweet and more texturally palatable. They are best made fresh but can be stored for months if all parts of the petal are carefully covered. They lose some flavour and colour and become harder with storage.

1 scented (unsprayed) rose, picked on a dry day   100g (4oz / ½ cup) caster sugar

1 egg white

Baking parchment

Very clean paint brush or pastry brush

Shake the rose to get rid of bugs, then remove all the petals.
   Whisk the egg white very slightly to break it up.
   Pour the sugar into a shallow dish.
   Paint the petals thoroughly with egg white, tilting to make sure that it looks shiny all over – front and back – but not dripping. Drop the petal into the sugar, spoon more sugar over the top of it. Shake off excess sugar, make sure the whole petal is covered. Put onto the baking parchment to dry – they should be ready to use in half an hour. If you are wanting to store them for longer dry overnight on the baking parchment before putting into a storage container.
   Other flowers that crystallise well include primroses and violets.

ROSE GERANIUM SCENTED SUMMER BERRIES

This is my favourite way to eat berries in the summer. Gather an abundance of berries for this dish, a mixture of whatever is bountiful: strawberries, raspberries, loganberries, blueberries, blackberries, gooseberries, black-, white- or redcurrants…
   The heady scent of rose geranium enhances the natural perfume of summer berries. Rose geranium *(Pelargonium graveolens)* is a pretty straightfor-

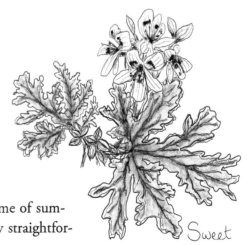

Sweet
Geranium

ward plant to grow in a pot – this from someone who is not known for her abilities in keeping pot plants alive. Keep the plant outside in summer and bring it into your bathroom or kitchen for the winter. Its leaves are fabulous for a quick pick-me-up – just brush your fingers along the leaves as you pass by. Or pick a couple of leaves and put them into your bath with a handful of rose petals for instant indulgence.

If you want to use less sugar in this recipe, add sweet cicely leaves, which add a **natural** sweetness.

Lucy

Scented geranium leaves and flowers   Sugar, agave or stevia to taste

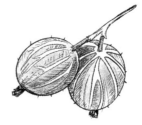

Heat the sugar, scented geranium leaves, a splash of water and any hard-skinned berries and currants until the sugar is dissolved and the fruit has softened. Take off the heat and stir through the strawberries, raspberries and other soft fruit and leave to cool. Decorate with fresh scented geranium leaves and flowers and a scattering of jasmine flowers if you have them. Serve with whipped cream or ice cream, perhaps along with a slice of lemon drizzle cake or a chocolate brownie.

Kitchen Witch Magic

Geranium: for love, protection, healing and prosperity.
Jasmine: for love and passion.

RASPBERRY AND ROSEWATER ETON MESS

This is one of the most heavenly desserts you are ever likely to eat – if you like rose and cardamom, that is, not everyone does! Light and airy meringues and cream scented with the exotic flavours of rose and cardamom transport you to a different dimension. The first place I tried this revamp of a classic British dessert was at Dishoom – a Bombay restaurant, now an institution – on a trip to London. I was evangelical about it and knew I had to figure out how to make it as soon as I got home, as I wasn't going to be able to live with only eating it once every couple of years.

It is simple to make – if you don't consider yourself a cook, or find yourself with surprise dinner guests, this is the dessert for you – buy your cream already whipped, your rosewater in a bottle, your cardamom pre-ground and your meringues pre-made. Or you can use the rosewater and crystallised rose petals you made from the previous recipes, and homemade meringues piped from a bag streaked with pink food colouring.

Lucy

How many this feeds depends on greed! I would suggest it serves 4.

4 medium sized meringues – homemade or bought

500ml (1 pint / 2½ cups) whipped cream

1 tablespoon caster sugar (optional depending how sweet-toothed you are!)

1 teaspoon rosewater

Cardamom seeds, from four pods, crushed (or ¼ teaspoon ground)

200g (7oz / 2 cups) raspberries (strawberries and pomegranate seeds are also lovely)

Optional: crystallised or fresh rose petals, pomegranate seeds, chopped unsalted pistachios to decorate

Crush the meringues in your hands, making sure you retain lots of bigger chunks, you don't just want powder.

Whip the cream until thick, go easy as it thickens so that you don't take it too far and turn it to butter. Remember you will be stirring in other ingredients, so don't overwork it.

Stir in the other ingredients, squishing some of the fruit to release its juices, turning the whole dessert a beautiful streaked pink and white. Taste and add more cardamom or rose if you like, but do it little by little, both are strong flavours and soapy if there is too much.

This is beautiful served with the flower shortbread cookies, decorated with crystallised rose petals, to which you can add some crushed cardamom seeds, fresh pomegranate seeds and chopped pistachios.

Kitchen Witch Magic

Meringues: light and joyful, connected to the Air element.
Cardamom: connected to love and the Water element.
Roses and raspberries: linked to love and the sacred feminine.

It is thought that to dream of Raspberries betokens success, happiness in marriage, fidelity in a sweetheart, and good news from abroad.

Plant Lore, Legends, and Lyrics by Richard Folkard

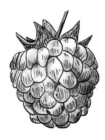

Porridge?!

In middle school we had a small garden in the corner of the concrete playground, and it was here that my friend Ruth said I should eat the blue flowers called "porridge". I did, I remember them tasting sweet. But we were promptly taken to the headteacher's office and told off "for being silly with flowers". The school even phoned my mum about the incident! As the only time I, a very anxious child, ever made it to the headteacher's office for a telling off, it became a pretty negative core memory. Many years later I would see a picture of those blue flowers, and realise the word my friend had said was "borage". These star-shaped blue flowers are completely edible and look lovely scattered over salads, cocktails or to top smoothie bowls (which aged eight or so, I wish I'd known, as I was made to believe I'd done something rather terrible and foolish).

Borage

Sarah

Midsummer's Light Simmer Pot

In summer we celebrate the longest day of the year. The sun's light has reached its peak and most of our time is spent outdoors in these months. The blend is cooling, fruity, and refreshing when we are trying to beat that summer heat. This pot reminds us to revel in the warming light of summer while calling forth intentions of joy, positivity and happiness.

Sarah Napoli

Water that has been charged by the sun.

St. John's Wort for blocking negativity.

Elderflower for grounding.

Rose for loving energy.

Oranges for positivity.

Lemons for happiness and rejuvenation.

Combine your ingredients. Stir clockwise and say:

Midsummer's rays radiant and bright,
Bring forth my intentions with
the warmth of your light.

Allow to simmer as long as desired and add water as needed.

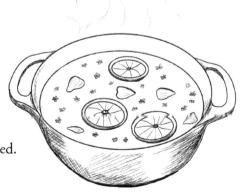

LATE SUMMER

DEEP SUMMER

Deep summer, I find, offers an opportunity to look around to see what flourishes of its own accord, to see what grows without tending, to see what rises wild and unfettered from the natural conditions in which it thrives.

Sometimes as humans we become used to controlling as much of the world and ourselves as we can. Sometimes we get focused on what we can cultivate, grow and intentionally tend. So focused on this conscious tending may we be, that we may even rip up or destroy or change what is naturally growing in our own little ecosystem, our own little biome, what is growing right where we are. We may even pull it up and put something else in its place that we think is prettier, or nicer, or even more beneficial or useful. I encourage us to consider summer as a time in which to pause, appreciate and look at, savor and explore, learn about and discover, what really grows right where you are, what thrives right where you stand, without the need for you to manipulate or control or change it.

I invite you to also consider how this might apply to the growing and thriving in your own personal life. How or what are you perhaps trying to manipulate or change or control in yourself or with the people in your life? Perhaps it is time to take a step back, to sit back, and to see what is already growing. What is already there? What is thriving in your world? What is thriving for you that doesn't require wrestling with or changing or trying to make it fit in a certain way? I encourage you to soften and see. Perhaps the mulberry trees are green and spreading in your world. Perhaps the clover is in bloom. Perhaps there are daisies. Perhaps there are monarch butterflies still bravely persistent on the milkweed in the field. Perhaps there are wild onion scapes, with their little purple heads. Perhaps there is yarrow, white and waiting, and interwoven in its own curious way with the health of your own blood and body. Perhaps that project that sings your name is waiting for you to pause to see it.

Molly Remer

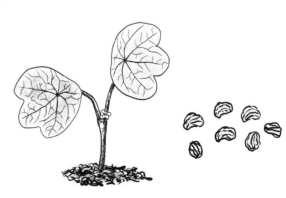

Summer Pickled Vegetables

This is a simple and ancient method of food preservation. It is a brilliant way to preserve the bounty of summer and to get through a long winter.

Chopping, salting and packing vegetables into vessels would be done as a community to preserve a glut. They would be packed into a watertight vessel, layered with salt, allowing beneficial microbes to do their thing, changing the sugars and starches in the vegetables into acids that preserve the whole. It is an interesting project in allowing and trusting the process, passed down from generation to generation through the millennia.

There is something beautifully meditative about standing in front of a pile of cabbage and methodically slicing, salting and packing it into a jar, knowing that in a few weeks it will be transformed into something quite different. There is a great satisfaction in lining up completed jars, knowing they're there for a later date.

A wonderful way to do this, and to make light work of it, is to get a group of like-minded magical friends together and make a fun day of it. All these jobs would have been communal once upon a time. The same goes with any creative process. There's healing to be had from this and it seems to magnify the medicine in the food itself.

This is alchemy.

This recipe is great because you can swap out the carrots for pretty much any vegetable, cut chunky. All root veg ferment particularly well, radishes, chunks of cabbage… (potatoes may be the only vegetable that I wouldn't recommend!)

Cucumbers need to be small and kept whole, courgettes work well when they're small, cauliflower works particularly well, broken into small florets. Peppers add a lovely splash of colour, whole cherry tomatoes become little fizz bombs that pop as you bite into them.

The onion and garlic are important as they add delicious flavour.

The flavours are changed into a sour and tangy crunchy pickle. A gut-healing, digestion-stimulating, crunchy condiment infused with the flavours of the garlic and herbs.

Penny Allen

450g (1lb) carrots or a mix of vegetables	Juice of 1 lemon
50g (2oz) onion	400ml (14fl oz) water
3 cloves of garlic	10 peppercorns
Sprigs of fresh dill, marjoram, basil or mint	15g (1 tablespoon) sea salt

1 litre (2 pint / 1 quart) Kilner jar

Cut carrots into thin sticks lengthways or pretty flower shapes if you're feeling whimsical. Peel and cut the onion into chunks, peel and thinly slice the garlic cloves. Pack all the vegetables tightly into the jar. Laying the jar on its side makes this job easier. Make sure there is about 5cm / 2in of space at the top of the jar as the liquid will need to cover the vegetables fully.

Add the salt into the water and stir until dissolved. Pour lemon juice into the jar and then follow with the salted water. Fill to above the vegetables but below the top level of the jar, leaving about 3cm / 1¼in from the top. This should be enough water to just barely cover the vegetables. Importantly, I add a weight onto the top of the veg to keep them submerged when the lid is clipped shut. This is key to the process so that the vegetables are fully submerged under the brine. We want to exclude air to encourage the lactobacillus bacteria (anaerobes) who create a wonderful acidic environment. They do this by digesting the sugars and starches in the veg and converting them into beneficial acids. I use a small jam jar or a couple of glass weights, purpose-made for this process. Clip the lid on tight.

Sit the jar on a countertop at room temperature somewhere out of the way. Allow to ferment with the lid closed for 2 weeks at least. You might hear gases escaping through the orange seal. This is great. This means fermentation is taking place successfully. I like to sit the jar on a plate or bowl as sometimes some of the liquid will also escape the seal.

The best way to know when these are ready is by tasting them. They should have a mouth-watering, fresh, tangy, sour flavour.

You can enjoy these just as finger food from the jar, dipped into something like hummus or home-made garlic mayo. Cut a couple of them finely and mix through a salad. Construct an antipasto board with the pickled veg as the perfect accompaniment. Cut finely and add to a toasted sandwich. Table-spoons of the brine itself are brilliant added to a vinaigrette, or to mayonnaise, even taken as a 'good gut shot' first thing in the morning on an empty stomach! A tablespoon swirled into soup or chicken broth is delicious.

From a health perspective you don't need heaps of these a day, a couple of fermented carrot sticks or even a teaspoon of the brine adds so many beneficial microbes to your digestive system. These foods stimulate our digestive system, adding beneficial microbes to our gut, which cleanse and detox us. A teaspoon of a fermented veg once a day is enough to change your gut health for the better, but obviously you can eat them in larger quantities if you feel drawn.

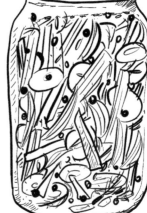

   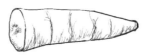

Asian Slaw

My step-grandmother Kim Vo was from Vietnam and fled to Europe during the Vietnam war. A woman of tiny stature, she made food with the most incredible flavour – we still make her Vietnamese pork stew on a monthly basis and remember her with love. This slaw has the flavours of *nuoc mam,* the staple Vietnamese condiment, which I learned to love, thanks to her (to make this simply omit the oils). With a distinctive funky tang from the fermented fish sauce, lemon or lime for sourness, sugar for sweetness, chilli for heat and garlic for punch, it is magic in a jar, transforming the simplest bowl of steamed white rice into a feast. We have this slaw so often, but it is different each time depending on the veggies we have to hand. It is stunning with any Thai or Vietnamese dish, but just as good beside roast chicken, barbecued meat or sticky ribs.

If you are preparing the slaw in advance, do not add the herbs or dressing until you are about to serve.

Lucy

Serves 4

Finely shredded vegetables – ½ cabbage (red or white), 2 grated carrots. A couple of spring onions (scallions), chopped

A handful each of mint and coriander, chopped

Optional extras include shredded radishes, sticks of cucumber, tiny broccoli or cauliflower florets, bean sprouts, shredded snow peas (mangetout), grated apple (add squeezed lemon to prevent browning)

Dressing

Juice of one lime

Two teaspoons fish sauce (Thai or Vietnamese *nam plaa, not* oyster sauce)

1 teaspoon sugar

Half a bird's eye chilli, finely chopped

1 small clove of garlic, finely chopped or grated

2 tablespoons sunflower, canola, vegetable or peanut oil

1 teaspoon toasted sesame oil (optional)

50g (2oz) roasted, salted, skinless peanuts, roughly chopped

Prepare all the vegetables, place in a large bowl and toss to mix. Combine the ingredients for the dressing and adjust to taste. Add herbs and pour over the vegetables just before serving. Toss well.

Top with a handful of chopped peanuts, if using.

Kitchen Witch Magic

Carrots: for fertility, positive energy and clarity.
Peanuts: for energy and creation.
Chillies: bring fire, energy, strength and passion.

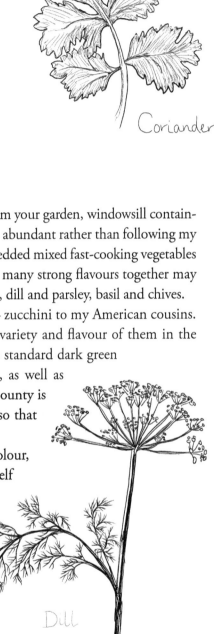

Coriander

SUMMER'S BOUNTY FRITTERS

This is a celebration of summer's bounty, be that collected from your garden, windowsill containers, allotment, local farm-shop, market or store. Use what is abundant rather than following my ingredients slavishly. You need two cups of grated/finely shredded mixed fast-cooking vegetables and ⅓ cup chopped herbs. Be thoughtful about your choices as too many strong flavours together may clash. Herb combinations that tend to work are: coriander and mint, dill and parsley, basil and chives.

The vegetables that speak to me most of summer are courgettes – zucchini to my American cousins. Though you can get them all year round now, nothing beats the variety and flavour of them in the summer. Our local farm shop sells such a selection. As well as the standard dark green ones, there are yellow – my favourite – green and white striped, as well as yellow and green patty pan squashes. If you grow your own their bounty is magnificent, though you do have to work to keep up with them so that they don't turn to woody marrows!

This dish is a celebration of summer on a plate: a riot of colour, freshness, zing and flavour. It is my go-to lunch that I make myself to eat in the sunshine, or as a quick starter for a last-minute summer dinner party. I serve them with a quick tomato salad, or a drizzle of tomato chilli jam (see next recipe).

Gathering the herbs is my favourite part of the whole thing. Each time I use a slightly different selection based on what is most abundant – but always several different kinds.

Lucy

Dill

Makes 8 – feeds 2 for lunch, 4 for starters

One medium courgette, grated (if you have access to fresh courgette flowers you can shred a couple of these as well)

One medium carrot, grated

5 green beans/runner beans/sugar snap peas, finely sliced

One spring onion (scallion), shallot or ¼ onion, cut into thin rounds

2 eggs

A big handful of fresh herbs, chopped (about ⅓ cup chopped) – coriander, dill, marjoram, oregano, mint, basil, chives, parsley, nasturtium flowers and leaves

4 tablespoons flour (gluten-free is fine)

100g (4oz) feta or goat's cheese

Salt and pepper

Extra virgin olive oil

Heat your largest frying pan (skillet) over a medium heat. Beat the eggs in a large bowl. Add all the vegetables and herbs, and the flour. Season well with salt and pepper. Stir till thoroughly combined. Crumble over the cheese and stir through gently. Add 2 tablespoons of olive oil to the pan. Blob a tablespoon of batter into the pan, you should fit four in a large frying pan. Flatten slightly. Fry on the first side for about 3 minutes until dark golden. Flip and fry for 2 minutes on the other side. Remove to a plate covered with kitchen paper to drain. Add more oil to the pan and fry the remaining batch of batter.

Drizzle with some tomato chilli jam or tomato salsa and a sprinkling of chopped herbs or herb flowers.

Kitchen Witch Magic

If you have ever grown courgettes in your garden, you'll know the plant can be very abundant, so it can be used spells for increase, abundance and prosperity.

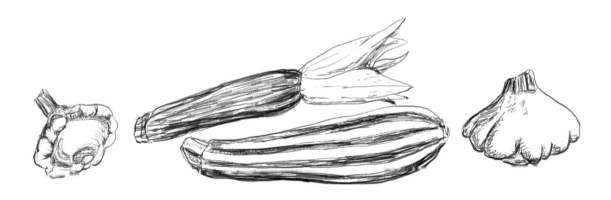

Tomato Chilli Jam

This is a recipe that my stepmother learned from a demo at the Ballymaloe Cookery School and made each year throughout most of my childhood. I in turn now do the same, when the local glasshouse and farm shop discount the prices on their bounty of super-ripe tomatoes. It is quick to make and super sweet – hence the name! It is also very runny, more sauce-like than thick chutney. We use it as a flavoursome replacement for shop-bought sweet chilli sauce – it has the same impact, more chilli flavour rather than chilli heat and a big sticky sweet hit. It has a beautiful East-meets-West vibe, with chillies, garlic, ginger and my favourite seasoning – *nam plaa* – fish sauce. If you're not sure you like it, just add half quantities: it adds a savoury, almost smoky, tang to the sauce. If you want to make it vegan, replace the fish sauce with salt.

This keeps for well over a year, though we've usually eaten our way through our batch by Christmas.

Serve with cheese and crackers, drizzle over fish cakes or potato cakes, burgers or grilled meats, an Asian chicken salad. Add it to homemade BBQ sauce and sticky marinades. Just about anything savoury and deep fried is sublime dipped into it: fried chicken, cheese croquettes, spring rolls, deep fried tofu or calamari…

Lucy

Makes 3 x 450ml / 1lb standard jam jars

3 fat mild red Dutch chillies (avoid spicy chillies like bird's eye or Scotch bonnet, unless you love it super-hot!)

5 cloves garlic

50g (2oz) fresh ginger

1kg (2.2lb) very ripe tomatoes

200ml (7fl oz / 1 scant cup) white wine vinegar

4 tablespoons *nam plaa* Thai/Vietnamese fish sauce (*not* oyster sauce)

500g (18oz / 2¼ cup) caster sugar

Purée half the tomatoes in a food processor, skins on. Remove any excess watery juice and seeds. Peel the ginger and garlic and take the tops off the chillies (and remove the seeds if you don't want it too spicy). Roughly chop and add to the blender.

Boil a kettle and fill a large bowl with the water. Make a cross on the bottom of the remaining tomatoes and leave in the water for about 1 minute until the skin starts to peel back. Remove from the water and carefully skin the tomatoes and chop in half. Remove and discard the core and seeds. Chop the flesh into ½cm / ¼in dice.

Put the purée, sugar, fish sauce and vinegar into a large pan and bring to the boil slowly, stirring so that it doesn't stick. Add the chopped tomatoes and simmer. Cook gently for 30–40 minutes, stirring every 5 minutes to prevent sticking.

When thickened, pour into sterilised glass jars. Allow to cool. Store in the fridge.

HERBS

Coriander, dill, fennel, marjoram, oregano, mint, basil, feverfew, chives, parsley, thyme, lovage, sweet cicely – summer is the time that herbs are in abundance. Just a tiny sprinkle of their pungent leaves adds vibrance to any dish.

Many of our recipes call for herbs, but kitchen witches use herbs in myriad other ways to purify and heal.

Making Herb Bundles for Burning

Smudging or saining is using the smoke from smouldering herbs to purify, cleanse or sanctify a sacred space, object, animal or person, it has been used in many cultures since the dawn of time.

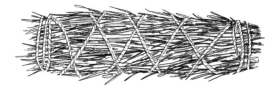

To make a herb bundle for burning, cut lengths (20–25cm / 8–10in) of woody aromatic herbs such as juniper, lavender, sage or rosemary. While still fresh, lay them in a bundle, tie one end tightly around the stems, you can lay rose petals on top. Then, starting at the bottom, wrap cotton thread or twine upwards around the bundle, tying the herbs tightly together. Once you reach the top, wrap downwards towards the stems and tie the thread off securely. Hang them up to dry out of direct sunlight for a full lunar month before use. You can use your saining stick for rituals, spells, ceremony or as gifts.

Drying Herbs

Harvest herbs in summer when they are at their peak, dry them for use throughout the rest of the year. Drying racks can be fashioned from scraps of wood. Screw hooks in like a little coat rack and attach to a wall or door – or if you find an actual coat rack in a thrift store, like the ones that hook over doors – you can repurpose them too! You can store these bundles hanging as they are or in jars (you can recycle suitably tall jars for this). Be sure to label your jars!

Tisanes

Tisane is a term for a medicinal drink or infusion using herbs, spices, flowers and/or leaves, it can be applied to any herbal infusions that don't use actual tea leaves. They are made by simply steeping fresh or dried ingredients in a teapot to extract their properties. If using herbs straight from your garden give them good shake or a rinse under the tap first. Steep a handful of the herb in boiling hot water for about 10 minutes, strain and drink – sweeten with honey if you like. You can also chill them and serve over ice, perhaps with a drizzle of honey.

You can buy most of the herbs mentioned below dried and loose – or ready to go in teabags if that is easier for you – from health food shops.

If you are pregnant, breastfeeding or taking medications always check first with a qualified herbalist before taking herbs. Be aware that not all parts of a plant may be safe to consume, and plants may be easily mistaken for others. If you are uncertain always seek further advice.

Simple Tisane Recipes

Chamomile – Soothing and comforting, chamomile tea is used to calm the nervous system and bring restful sleep. The white daisy-like flowers are the parts usually used to make tea. It is particularly lovely with a spoonful of honey.

Dandelion – You can make dandelion tea from the leaves, flowers, or roots. Sarah's favourite is using the flowers – add a handful into a teapot to steep and add half a lime or lemon too. Enjoy it hot or chilled over ice. The leaves are associated with the urinary tract – reflected in one of its traditional folk names "piss-a-bed", it acts as a powerful diuretic. It eases menstrual symptoms, cholesterol issues and supports breastfeeding.

Honeysuckle – (Flowers only, the black berries are toxic) is used to soothe the throat and respiratory tract and soothe the stomach, it is anti-inflammatory and helps boost the immune system. A syrup made from the flowers was traditionally used as a cough syrup. The flower buds are rich in salicylic acid – the painkilling compound used to make aspirin – so it is good for easing aches and pains. It is delicious served diluted over ice. Honeysuckle has a sweet floral almost vanilla flavour and is a beautifully soothing tea to drink, you can feel your nervous system relaxing as you sip it.

Honeysuckle

Honeysuckle was the first thing I ever grew... albeit unintentionally. Aged four I picked up a bare twig off the garden path to mark where I had planted seeds in my little garden. The seeds didn't come up, but the stick came to life and flourished into a honeysuckle bush, growing as fast as Jack's beanstalk. The Chinese refer to it as "the herb of immortality" because of its ability to flourish, however hard it is cut back. I can see why!
Lucy

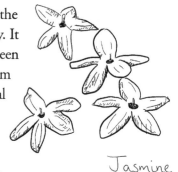
Jasmine

Jasmine – Known in India as "Queen of the Night" and "moonlight of the grove", in Christianity the star-shaped flowers are associated with Mary. It is connected with feminine qualities of sweetness and love and has been used in women's health and healing for centuries for the nervous system and female reproductive system, to calm and soothe PMS, menstrual headaches and ease afterpains after birth. Antiviral and antibacterial it is settling on the stomach. The fresh flowers can be used to make tea, or added to cooling drinks. Jasmine tea – black tea with jasmine flowers or oil added – is readily available to buy from Chinese supermarkets and health food shops and is often served with *dim sum* or after a meal.

Lady's Mantle – The botanical name of this powerful plant is *Alchemilla* derived from the word "alchemy" and it is known by such lovely folk names as the "little alchemist" or "little magical one" because it was favoured by alchemists who believed it to possess magical and healing properties. The dew drops that collect on the leaves were used in alchemical potions, as well as by women to promote beauty. Teas made from the leaves have been used to support the womb, bring on contractions and help with heavy bleeding after birth and around the menopause for generations.

Lemon Balm and Lemon Verbena – Both these herbs have a strong lemony scent and flavour and pair well together. Lemon verbena is more subtle flavoured shrub that hates frost, whereas lemon balm, a member of the mint family, is bold in its flavour and spreads like mint – you'll never be rid of it, though it does die back in winter. Calming and soothing, lemon balm *(Melissa officinalis)* has been used for centuries to lift the spirits and ease the mind. A lovely summer tea, it acts well to support digestion after a heavy meal.

Raspberry Leaf – Has been used for centuries to prepare the uterus for birth in the last month of pregnancy and help to soothe and tone it postpartum. It is also used premenstrually to soothe the womb. Add in hibiscus flower for a rich red colour for moon time healing.

Rosemary – Has been used medicinally since at least ancient Egyptian times. Among its many benefits, rosemary can help open the airways and calm the mind.

Lemon Verbena

My favourite herb to use in rituals is rosemary: it has cleansing and healing properties, it celebrates memory, it can soothe a sore throat, and bring peace to a troubled mind. It also cooks nicely into a range of dishes – and is an easy herb to work with, as it grows well in a pot, and is fairly hardy. One of the easiest ways to use rosemary is to take it as a tea with honey, to soothe an overstimulated mind and promote healing when you are run down. I find that adding rosemary to a bath is a beautiful way to relieve sore sinuses, too.

Alice Tarbuck

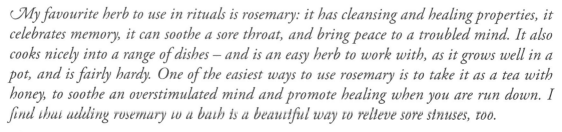

Valerian

Valerian tea has been used as a traditional medicine as far back as ancient Greek and Roman times, and in my family it has been used as a remedy against stress, anxiety and insomnia for generations.

One cup of pure valerian root tea before bed helps to relax the brain, thus helping with those endless scenarios swimming around your head in the middle of the night. For my teenage son, one cup of it helps him focus by numbing the panic of the anxiety attack. Combined with breathing techniques the tea has been a life-saver more than once. For my youngest, a small cup of the tea with a little bit of honey has him back asleep until the morning time with no recollection of the nightmare.

If anyone of us is feeling under the weather, has a sore throat and needs rest, I mix the valerian tea with a few drops of propolis.

Indra Roelants

Vervain – *Verbena officinalis* is often combined with valerian to make a calming, sleep-inducing tea. Vervain is useful for migraine, depression, nervous exhaustion and those who overwork.

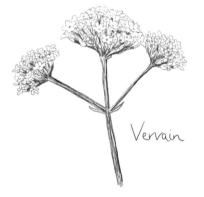

It was considered sacred, a wizard's herb for casting spells and a vital ingredient in magic potions… the Druids used it to clean their altars.

Healing with Flowers, **Anne McIntyre**

Vervain

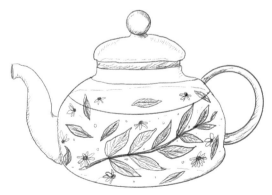

MEDICINE SPOON SPELL

The Medicine Spoon Spell is a spell for healing. If you have had an argument, are seeking to reconnect estranged friends or family or are feeling internal conflict – such as seeking to break up with diet culture and calorie counting – gathering around the kitchen table is often a good place to start. These things are not by any means easy, but this ritual will help support the process.

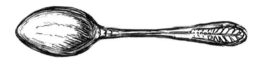

☾ Start a simple simmer pot of herbs connected to healing: sage, rosemary, lavender, rose and mint are all suitable, and one sliced lemon.

☾ Let it simmer for half an hour. In this time you maybe want to meditate, reflect, journal on the situations and if possible reflect on empathy for each person involved.

☾ Turn off the hob and let the simmer pot cool. This time can be used to shower or bath with the intention of washing away any lingering resentment, hurts and/or anger.

☾ Now wash all your cutlery (knives, forks, spoons – so that anyone eating in this kitchen will be connected to this healing magic) in the simmer pot water, rinse with clean water and put away, but save one spoon – this our medicine spoon for this spell.

☾ Lay the spoon down somewhere clean – this might be your kitchen table, altar or windowsill.

☾ Light three candles beside it – they represent the past, present, future. As you light each candle:

  ☆ Reflect on the past: what hurts have occurred, for yourself but also how others may feel.

  ☆ Reflect on the present: the situation as it stands

  ☆ Reflect on the future: what you may need to do to move forward – does the situation require forgiveness? Compromise? Acceptance?

☾ Take a moment with the candles burning and when you are ready with intention, blow them out saying: "Whatever is past may we release it, whatever is present may we learn from it, and whatever is future may we look forward to creating it."

☾ And with this decisive action we set an intention, a step, however small towards healing: can you send a message, make a phone call, arrange a date in the diary?

☾ Finally, place this spoon into bowl of sugar or honey and use it in some way to continue the healing gesture in this kitchen, such as:

☆ Baking cookies as a gift

☆ Inviting someone round for a cup of tea

☆ Keeping it on the table to serve sugar with coffee or tea at the end of a meal, or to top breakfast pancakes or French toast.

☾ Close the ritual by saying: "May the situation be sweetened, and hearts softened."

BLESSING

It is a blessing to be. It is a blessing to be here. It is a blessing to be here now. It is a blessing to be here now together.

Veronika Robinson

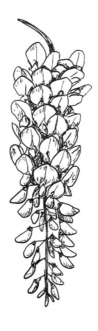

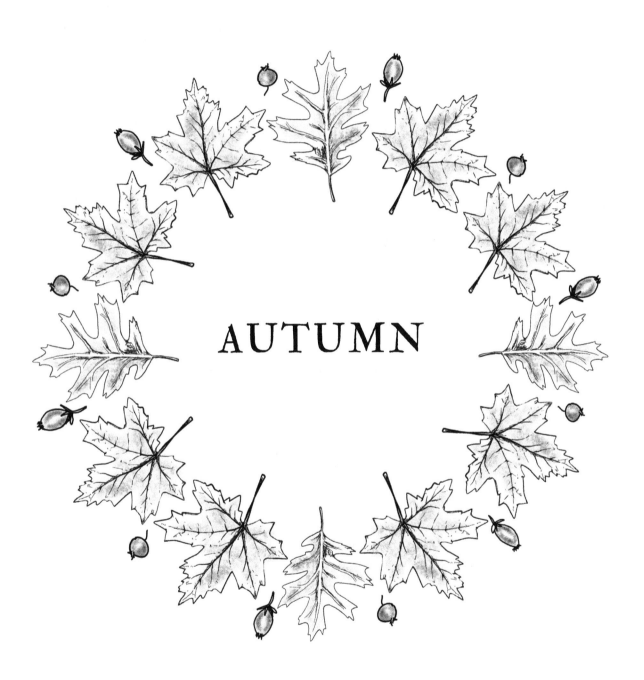

AUTUMN

Roasted nuts, chutneys and pickles, succulent squashes, slow roasted meats, freshly foraged mushrooms and orchard fruits – they make the ingredients for rich and warming autumnal dishes. This was a time when our ancestors would hunt and stock up on meat for the coming cold weather. The leaves turn, their colours of red, yellow, browns and purples are mirrored in rosehips, apples, medlars, elderberries, sloes and haws. The harvest is a time of hard work and joyful play; once this time would have seen great gatherings for the harvest and people coming together to do the most important farm jobs of the year to see communities through the winter.

Fall is a time of many harvest festivals: Lughnasadh, Summer's End, the Autumn Equinox, mushroom hunts, nut gathering, blackberry picking expeditions, and of bonfires, for Halloween, Samhain, Bonfire Night, as well as Day of the Dead *(Dia de Los Muertos)*, All Souls… it is a time to surrender to the darker season and step into the winter with warmth in your heart.

KITCHEN TABLE CHARMS

Arrange twigs of coppery beech leaves and dancing silver coins of *Lunaria* (honesty) in a jar. Pumpkins and squashes carved as lanterns (the flesh of which can later be turned into velvety soups).

Corn dollies made of corn stalks, you may be able to gather a few stalks whilst out walking by fields and meadows.

A bowl of freshly harvested apples.

Autumn Craft

A Kitchen Witch! Of course we couldn't leave out this hanging hag charm of the Kitchen Witch – a poppet or doll traditionally placed in kitchens for good luck. The Kitchen Witch was once thought to prevent kitchen mishaps and ward off mischievous spirits. She often rides a broom, a wooden spoon, a whisk or other kitchen implement. Those called witches would have hung charms of herbs and sigils in kitchens for centuries, and these modern poppets connect the magic of the witch and her protection magic. You may buy one or make your own!

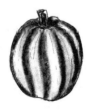

Seasonal Meditation: Autumn

This meditation is perfect for a quiet dark autumnal evening. Please be aware that it does mention – gently – ideas of loss and grief, so be compassionate with yourself if you are feeling these emotions very strongly at present, or save this meditation for a time that you feel is right for you.

Close your eyes and relax as we settle and breathe.

As the last golden light of the sun sets on a late autumn evening, you walk through a woodland that is resplendent in caramel shades of rich browns, yellows and oranges. Leaves fall from branches, dancing around you as you walk and falling underfoot. You catch the scent of wood smoke in the air, and deep rich forest smells of moss and earth and damp leaves.

You arrive at your destination: a wooden house in the woods. It is simple in design but strong. Light glows from every window, inviting you closer. You slip through the front door and find yourself standing in a great wooden room. Like many ancient barns, the ceiling is tall and beams arch overhead. Autumnal leaves have been gathered into great garlands to hang from the beams.

A long table stands proud in the middle of this large room. It is abundant with food and treasures of the season. The great table is decorated with pumpkins of every size and colour, each holding a glowing candle in its belly – they have been carved with faces, animals and imagery from nature – trees, clouds, suns and moons. Around the pumpkins swaths of leaves in every autumnal hue are spread out in great blankets.

People are quietly carrying glass flagons of deep rich liquids: damson gin, blackberry wine and elderberry wine. Placed on the table, they shine richly in the lantern light. Others bring cakes made of apple and cinnamon still warm from the oven that scent the air. Still more people arrange cheeses and chutneys, steaming bowls of soups and stews with chunks of warm bread, biscuits made with nuts of the season, crunchy and sweet. And they hold out their hands for you to join them: *come now, gather, be warm!*

Once a feast on Samhain night might be called a "dumb supper" – a silent meal to honour those no longer with us. In honour of this you gather quietly, with a peacefulness and respect, lighting candles in golden holders.

When all is ready, the group gather around this table and raise a glass to those we have lost who join us here at this table in memory. The light of the sun in the Wheel of the Year stands in the west, where the sun sets: this is a time of farewell and gratitude for the summer and year, the harvest and memories that have blessed us.

With your respects now offered, the group begins to speak, each sharing stories of those lost and loved. Bringing them back to life with words and stories on this night of respect and of remembering.

Pause with this image

Take your time to journey from this meditation. Take some deep breaths, stretch, and allow yourself to sit with any grief or loss you are feeling. When you feel ready you may want to light a candle which you can blow out after a minute or put somewhere safe and supervised to burn through the evening and cast its light into the autumnal night.

EARLY AUTUMN

If spring is the season of the gardener, then fall is the season of the kitchen witch, the time of year when the knife becomes a magic wand, the work of turning the harvest into medicine, nutrition and things that can sustain us over the coming months.

Melissa Jayne Madara, Missing Witches: Mabon 2022

GATHERING – BLACKBERRYING

Blackberrying is a family tradition that I'm assuming goes back multiple generations – parents, grandparents and children and friends gather with pots for berries, sticks for pulling down brambles, thick trousers and boots. We marvel at the bounty glistening in the hedges, the biggest juiciest berries always just out of reach, of course. We fill our pots and our bellies too. Then head home to make a quick batch of blackberry jam whilst the scones are baking. We eat together around the table, butter melting on the still-hot scones, jam dripping down our already purple fingers.

Lucy

ELDERBERRY AND BLACKBERRY SYRUP

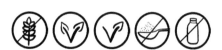

Elderberry

Elderberries are packed with antioxidants and vitamins. They also contain a compound proven to fight cold and flu viruses, reducing the length of illness and severity of symptoms. In England and Ireland there is an abundance of these sprays of tiny jewel-like berries in the hedges every September, but you have to get there before the birds. Green elderberries and the green stems have toxins in them so be sure to remove them. It is safest to eat elderberries cooked as when eaten raw they can cause stomach ache and nausea. They have a very distinctive flavour which I am personally on the fence about, hence why I add blackberries to my syrup as well. Be sure to check the centre of each blackberry when picking to make sure it is white-ish green: a discoloured brown or juicy centre lets you know the maggots have got there first.

  Both fruits are high in vitamin C, so this is a great tonic to see you through the winter. You can take a teaspoonful each morning as a preventative, or at the first sign of a sniffle. It's also nice drizzled over plain yogurt or made into a cordial over iced water or with hot water and an extra squeeze of lemon and perhaps a few drops of echinacea tincture to give your immune system a boost (see my ImmuniTea recipe later in the book.)

Extra berries can be slowly dried in a very low oven and used like raisins, or frozen.

Lucy

Makes about 600ml (1 pint / 2¾ cups)

450g (1lb) combination of freshly picked elderberries and blackberries

350g (12oz / 1½ cups) caster sugar

Juice of one lemon

Remove the elderberries from the stalks (I use a fork to strip them off, a trick that works fabulously well for currants too!). Discard any hard green elderberries. Put both types of berries into a saucepan and add the water. Simmer for 15 minutes or until the berries are soft.

Strain through a piece of muslin or a very fine plastic sieve and return it to the pan. Add the sugar and the lemon juice, stirring until dissolved. Bring back to the boil for about 10 minutes, allow to cool before pouring through a funnel into sterilised bottles. Screw the lids on and store in a cool, dry place.

Kitchen Witch Magic

Elder: known as a tree of protection. The word elder is thought to connect to 'aeld' the Anglo-Saxon word for fire. Correspondence tables often connect the berries and flowers to the element of Air. Between these two elements, of Air and Fire – we have an energy of rising heat and stoking fires, exactly what is needed to boost immunity.

Blackberries: associated with the supernatural, with old folks in Ireland still shouting warnings to leave them be after the end of September (or for others this is the end of October), because you will be taken by the fairies/the devil has pissed on them/they are for the witches. Consider yourself warned!

Blackberry

FORAGING: MEDLARS

Alice Tarbuck

During one of the pandemic years, I entered a silent war with an invisible foe, over the medlar tree on my dog walk. It is a small tree, its branches narrow. For all its youth, however, it does fruit. Not a great many medlars appear on the tree, but enough to make two or three small harvests. Every day, I would walk past that tree – as it came into bud, as it put forth its pretty white flowers, and then, as the year ripened, its strange fruiting bodies.

Medlar fruits are neither pretty, nor widely eaten these days. The medlar, or *Mespilus germanica,* is a small tree in the *Rosaceae* family, and has been grown for its fruits since Roman times. The fruits have a number of colourful names, due to their appearance, such as the Middle English, 'open-arse'! These names, and the strange fruit they refer to, may dissuade the contemporary consumer, but it seems more likely to be the process by which they become edible.

Medlars are high in tannins, and this means that, even when 'ripe', they are extremely bitter. In order to be rendered edible, they must be 'bletted' before they are eaten. What does 'bletting' refer to? Well, simply put, they must be allowed to freeze and then rot. This usually happens by leaving medlar fruit on the tree until the first frost begins to break down the tannins inside them, and then picking them and allowing them to rot until their flesh ceases to be firm and bitter, and instead becomes custardy and sweet. Medlars can be eaten straight, like this, but are more usually made into jelly, to be eaten with cheese. Their historic popularity has waned, but it is still possible to buy medlar jams and jellies – they taste quite unlike any other fruit.

The fruits, however, are difficult to buy – even the unspeakably posh grocers' shops near me don't sell them – and so I passed this tree, every single day, guarding it with my sight. I didn't want all the fruit, you understand. Only enough to make a little pot of jelly. My covetous gaze might have acted as a protection spell, but my desire was clearly only one amongst many. I thought that I had detected something others would pass over, uncommented on. Arrogantly, perhaps, I had assumed that the residents who came through this scrap of parkland wouldn't see the wonder that was right in front of them.

However, pride comes before a fall. Many foragers are keen to share recipes, preserving tips, cautions against poison – far fewer, the locations where they find their bounty. It was, of course, impossible to keep this fruit-tree secret, and I was, it transpired, certainly not the only one who had spotted it. One day, long before the first frost – before Hallowe'en had even passed – I walked by the tree to find it bare. Whoever had chosen to harvest the medlars, they certainly hadn't done so responsibly, leaving some for those who came after them. The entire tree had been completely stripped.

During the pandemic, as we moved through uncertainties, changing restrictions, and the contortion of time, small things gained disproportionate significance. I was absolutely devastated by the loss of those medlars – not that they had ever been mine, really. I remember searching the tree, and the ground around it, looking for any they might have dropped. Whilst I don't know who took them, I hope they treated them properly – bletted them, made them into something that delighted them in those strange times. I forgive them – we were perhaps none of us at our most generous during a global pandemic – but I haven't forgotten the strange sting of it.

There are lessons here, of course – about hope, about sharing, and about responsible foraging, making sure you leave enough for others. But there are also lessons about vigilance, and timing. I am not perfect, you know. The following year… well. Of course, I didn't strip the tree, but let's not pretend that I don't have a little bag of medlars in the freezer! During summer, I will let them out to blett, and then make jelly for winter.

Medlars

ROWAN: KEEPER OF THE WINTER SPARK

Jacqueline Durban

One of my favourite edge-of-autumn exploits is gathering berries from the Hedge Hermitage garden rowan tree, a beloved friend. These rowan berries (although strictly speaking they are 'pomes'), aside from being full of vitamin C, help us keep our spark alight through the winter months, both through spoonfuls of syrup and the brightness of rowan berry threads draped in every possible nook and cranny.

Like my equally beloved blackberry, rowan is a member of the rose family. She is a mountain dweller, one of her folk names being 'The Lady of the Mountain'. Her berries are much loved by crows and other birds. Indeed, that is where her Latin name, *Sorbus aucuparia* comes from; *sorbus* meaning 'reddish-brown', which her common name 'rowan', from the Germanic, 'raud-inan', 'to redden', echoes. The second part of her Latin name, *aucuparia,* translates as 'bird catcher', and speaks of the liminal space that rowan often inhabits, the space where nature's generosity and beauty meet human cruelty and disconnection. 'Bird-catcher' comes from the practice of using her berries to bait and capture birds, an ancient practice sometimes still used today. Having such a close association with humans as a blessing and a protection, rowan has much to teach us about who we truly are.

But it was not just birds who were 'caught' by the rowan tree.

In Norse mythology the first woman was said to have come from a rowan tree and the tree is often deeply woven in with the feminine. In J.R.R. Tolkien's *The Two Towers,* the male Ents plant rowans to please the Entwives, and Quickbeam says of the rowan that, "no other people of the rose are so beautiful to me."

In the British Isles rowan has a long history of being used as a protection against witchcraft. A rowan tree grown close to the house was said to keep the home safe, and rowan sprigs were carried by people in their travels as equal armed crosses, bound with red thread and sewn into coat linings or popped into pockets. Rowan was also hung in barns and dairies to protect cows and dairy produce from enchantment. In 1597, James VI wrote about the use of rowan charms in his book *Daemonologie*. He noted that people protected their cattle against the evil eye by "knitting roun trees or sundriest kind of herbes to the haire and tails of the goods (animals)."

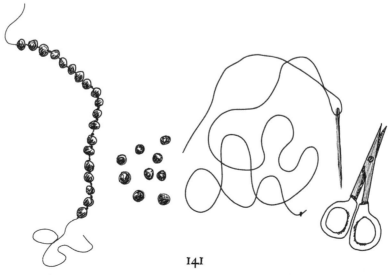

In spite of James VI's admonishments, one of my favourite seasonal rituals is to make my own rowan and red thread cross to protect our home on May Eve. As I weave, I marvel at the creamy froths of whipped up rowan blossom. That those delicate petals will become bunches of heavy red berries within a few months. And, in the late summer, I marvel that the heavy red berries were once delicate petals. An ordinary miracle. As I weave my rowan cross, I pray for my health, for the health of those I love and of the land. I feel the hands of my ancestors in mine as I work. Perhaps that in itself – to make deeper connection with those who knew that life and land are one – is the oldest and most precious prayer of all.

Although rowan was said to protect against witchcraft, her magic is much older than that. Her Anglo-Saxon name, *cwic-beám,* which became quickbeam/quicken-tree, had by the 19th century been misinterpreted as 'witch', hence 'witch tree' and 'wicken-tree'. As recently as 1618, Margaret Barclay was brought to trial for witchcraft in Scotland and burnt at the stake; one piece of evidence against her being that she carried a rowan twig tied with red thread in her pocket. It is as bitter as a rowan berry before frost to think that had she simply made her twig into a cross she may have escaped such punishment. How arbitrary our judgements of right and wrong truly are. How easily we condemn.

The traditions of the rowan are long-lasting and have much to teach us about the magic of the Earth and the people of the land. Like goddess-saint Brigid, whose sacred tree she is, she is strong enough to transcend changes in religion. Christianity is a faith woven through with trees: from the apple in Eden, to the burning bush, to the Cross. It is also entrenched in exploitative power, both of Church and State, which seeks through means of division to sever our connection to the Earth, to make us rootless, put out our fire, particularly the fire of the Feminine spirit. But rowan, like the Spirit, needs only the shallowest of soil to thrive, and to (mis)quote Paul Cudby in *The Shaken Path,* she reminds us that "every bush is burning". Rowan is able to thrive in the most seemingly adverse of circumstances, both extremes of temperature and rocky ground, just as we are sometimes called to do in this world of power imbalance and injustice. Whatever religion or spiritual path we might follow, we can reclaim that wilder fire and the right to thrive if we choose.

And so, in the late summer, I gather rowan berries in my basket, sure that each berry has a tiny flame inside it; a mindful preparation for turning from basking in the heat of the summer sun to attending to the small flame within as the months of winter dark beckon.

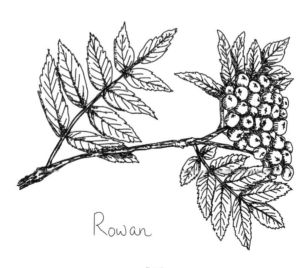

Rowan

Rowan Berry Winter Syrup

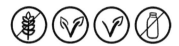

I like simple recipes, which I often make by feel, and so I invite you to feel your own way in making this.

Once gathered, I sort through, wash and freeze the berries overnight. Rowan berries shouldn't be eaten raw and are bitter to the taste, which is why the advice is to pick them after the first frost as that breaks them down a little and makes them sweeter. But these days our rowan berries are ripe long before the possibility of frost, and so using a freezer is a fine alternative and a way to mimic nature.

After a day or two, I defrost them and make a simple rowan berry preserve, or winter syrup, which I save to take a spoon of every morning through the winter months. Rowan berries are full of vitamin C, amongst other good things, and they help me stay in touch with my inner fire as I journey through the cold and dark. I love them! Often, I offer the last of our rowan berry syrup to the land even as the first spring green is buried under the snow. I know that the rowan berries will come again. It is an act of trust. This is how we make hope holy.

Jacqueline Durban

A basket of rowan berries

Just under the same amount of apples, peeled, cored, and diced. So, for example, if you have 1.3kg (3lb) of rowan berries, you will need 900g (2lb) of apples

Juice of 1 lemon

450g (1lb) of white sugar for every two cups of pulp produced by cooking the rowan berries and apples

25g (1oz) of chopped fresh ginger (optional)

Water

Sterilised jars

Put the rowan berries and apples into a stainless steel, glass, or ceramic pan. They should have room to boil.

Cover the fruit with cold water and bring to the boil over a medium heat. Simmer for 20 minutes or until the fruit is softened.

For a crystal clear jelly, let the mixture cool for a few minutes and then strain through a jam/jelly bag for at least 12 hours. Make sure not to squeeze the bag or your syrup will be cloudy. The straining is optional. I like to leave the fruit in mine, although it will keep better without.

Measure your strained liquid (or liquid and fruit) and weigh out the amount of sugar you need. Add both to a stainless steel, glass, or ceramic pan and simmer for around 10 minutes, or until the sugar has dissolved. Taste the mixture to see whether it's sweet enough. Rowan berries are bitter, and the taste can be surprising, so find a balance that you like. If you need to add more sugar, do that now and then simmer again.

Increase the heat and allow the mixture to boil for 5 minutes. You can test it to see if it's the consistency you'd like by putting a small plate in the freezer. Put a small amount of your syrup onto it, pop it back into the freezer for 1 minute and then push it with your finger. If it wrinkles then your syrup is done.

Pour the syrup into sterilised jars, seal, and label. It can be enjoyed with cheese, spread onto toast, or taken on a spoon as a winter tonic.

Kitchen Witch Magic

Rowan berries: anti-inflammatory, antibacterial and full of antioxidants, plus vitamins A and C. They are sacred to goddess-saint Brigid, who accompanies us through the winter months until we emerge with her at Candlemas (or Imbolc) at the beginning of February. They are trees of fire and help us to keep our inner flame alight through the winter.

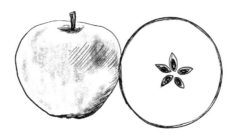

AUTUMN KOMBUCHA

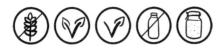

Kombucha is very dear to my heart as it was the first ferment I acquired many years ago and the positive effects it had on my body were astounding. I was very quickly hooked. There's a beauty to the rhythmic brewing of it, the cycle of making, the waiting, the harvesting, the making again, ad infinitum!

To make kombucha, it's best to first acquire a starter culture, or to be more precise, a scoby. This is just an acronym for Symbiotic Community of Bacteria and Yeast, a cellulose mat that grows to cover the surface of your brewing kombucha. This scoby is basically a piece of someone else's kombucha brew. (If you don't have a friend with one there are many options online to purchase.)

A cup of kombucha and a piece of scoby is enough to get you started. Each time you brew a batch, a new scoby is formed on the surface of the brew.

Kombucha lends itself beautifully to being flavoured with seasonal fruit, herbs and spices. We call this a 'second ferment'.

Penny Allen

750ml (1¼ pints / 3¼ cups) boiling water

2 teaspoons loose leaf tea or 2 teabags (green, white or black – organic is best)

150g (5oz / ¾ cup) organic caster sugar

1.2 litres (2 pints / 5 cups) room temperature filtered or bottled water

250ml (9fl oz / 1 cup) kombucha

1 kombucha scoby

3 litre (5 pint / 3 quart) Kilner jar or large Pyrex bowl or similar
Glass or plastic measuring jug (don't use a metal container when brewing kombucha)

Pour the boiling water into a jar, bowl or teapot and add 2 teaspoons of loose leaf tea or 2 tea bags (black, green or white tea all work well). Let this sit for a good few minutes to infuse and then strain into your brewing vessel.

Add the sugar and stir to dissolve.

Add the filtered water and stir again. The temperature of the sweetened tea should now be tepid and you should have just over 2 litres (3½ pints / 2 quarts) of liquid. If the liquid feels too warm, leave to stand for a few more minutes until it's a bit cooler.

Add the kombucha and the scoby.

Cover the jar with a clean cloth tied around with string or an elastic band. Don't be tempted to put a lid on it because the kombucha scoby needs air to thrive. (I also attach a label with the date.)

Put in a warmish place for a week to ten days (or 2 weeks in the colder months). It should be out of direct sunlight and somewhere it won't have to be moved. Use a spoon or a straw to take a taste after about day 7. I find day 10 is the perfect fermenting time for my taste buds. The taste you are looking for is a pleasing balance between sweet and sour.

Bottling

Lift off the culture (scoby) and put it in a bowl with 1 cup of your brewed kombucha and cover this with a plate or bowl just while you bottle the rest. This is going to be the starter for your next batch.

Pour the brewed kombucha into bottles through a funnel (it makes 2½ x 750ml bottles), or into another large Kilner jar. You can then store this in the fridge and enjoy as it is, or you can add something to flavour it and add extra nutritional benefits. It lends itself beautifully to being flavoured with berries of all sorts, rosehips, apple pieces, spices, herbs. I love to add foraged hedgerow plants to a brew – fabulous way to enjoy their medicine.

It's a very stable ferment and once it's bottled and in the fridge it keeps for weeks.

You don't need vast quantities of it to get the benefits. A small glass a day is loads.

Kitchen Witch Magic

Kombucha: contains all nine essential amino acids, B vitamins, and beneficial organisms. Very helpful in detoxification. It also helps digestion.

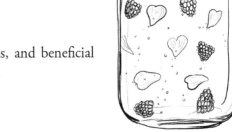

Sloe Gin

First you need to pick your sloes. Fruits of the blackthorn bush, in the British Isles they are abundant at the same time as blackberries and hawthorn. Like tiny plums, the size of a fat blueberry, they are a beautiful frosted purple blue. They're also bitter as hell! If you're tempted to try one raw, they turn your mouth inside out with bitterness! However, with lots of sugar, they add a beautiful colour and flavour to spirits to make a lovely homemade aperitif to sip on winter evenings before dinner with friends, or to add to cocktails, sparkling wine or water. Be careful when picking as the bushes are very spiky and you can easily get a nasty infection from these thorns. Be sure to clean and disinfect anywhere that you are pricked.

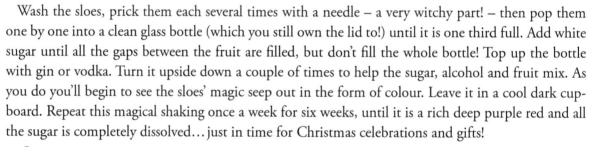

Sloe

Wash the sloes, prick them each several times with a needle – a very witchy part! – then pop them one by one into a clean glass bottle (which you still own the lid to!) until it is one third full. Add white sugar until all the gaps between the fruit are filled, but don't fill the whole bottle! Top up the bottle with gin or vodka. Turn it upside down a couple of times to help the sugar, alcohol and fruit mix. As you do you'll begin to see the sloes' magic seep out in the form of colour. Leave it in a cool dark cupboard. Repeat this magical shaking once a week for six weeks, until it is a rich deep purple red and all the sugar is completely dissolved…just in time for Christmas celebrations and gifts!

Lucy

Kitchen Witch Magic

Sloes: come from the blackthorn tree. Blackthorn has long been considered a magical tree. To some it's a witch's tree and anyone seen to carry a blackthorn walking stick might have been suspected of being a witch. In Celtic mythology, the blackthorn was considered to be a home to fairies and farmers would leave them well alone – even in the middle of a field! A fruit with magical connections indeed!

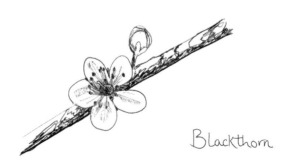

Blackthorn

Green Tomato Chutney

I share this recipe in honour of my ex-step-grandmother (on my English side): not everyone gets one of those in life! She was about as different to me as it's possible to get – tiny, neat, orderly, polite and very conservative. Every visit to her house was exactly the same, down to every item on the menu. She only made this one chutney. During childhood it seemed endless in its ubiquity, when all I really wanted was a jar of bought Branston Pickle. But now, as nostalgia tends to do, I find myself craving it, however it not being something you can buy, I have begun in my 40s to make it for myself and my family.

You're unlikely to be able to buy green tomatoes, except from a farm shop on request. If you grow tomatoes (which is simple to do in a tub or grow bag, even in the cool wet Irish climate, with the right variety you don't need a glasshouse), you'll always have lots to spare, especially when the weather is starting to turn autumnal but your tomato plants are still producing fruit. This is a great way to use them up and enjoy them through the colder months. It's fabulous with cold meats, toasted sandwiches, pasties and with cheese on crackers… or to give as a gift.

Lucy

300g (11oz) green tomatoes

1 medium cooking apple, peeled, cored

1 small onion

50g (2oz / ⅓ cup) sultanas

100g (4oz / ½ cup) light brown sugar

120ml (4fl oz / ½ cup) cider vinegar (or white wine vinegar)

1 teaspoon salt

1 tablespoon yellow mustard seeds

Peel the onion and dice it reasonably finely. Chop the tomatoes and apples into similar size cubes – no need to skin the tomatoes!

Combine all the ingredients in a saucepan and bring to a simmer uncovered. Stir frequently making sure it doesn't stick to the bottom or burn. Cook for 40 mins–1 hour until it is thick. Put into sterilised jars and cover. Store in a cool, dark place.

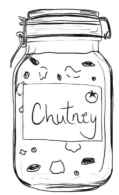

Kitchen Witch Magic

Tomato: early tomatoes were yellow and known in Europe as *pomi d'oro* – apples of gold and 'love apples' (and they were used in love and prosperity spells). Tomatoes are members of the deadly nightshade family – along with potatoes, chillis, peppers and aubergines (eggplant) which linked them in some people's minds to malefic magic and witches, as some nightshades could cause hallucinations. This also led to warding magic: a tomato on your mantelpiece was reputed to protect your home. In German folklore witches used nightshades to rouse werewolves – leading to the rather fabulous name 'wolf peach' for the tomato.

Onion: connected to Earth energy and protection, onions stuck with nails were used as warding charms in England.

Fig and Hazelnut Cake

Where there is cake, there is hope. And there is always cake.

Dean Koontz

  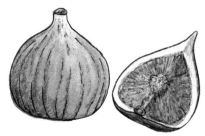

I have a thing for figs – their rich juicy taste of exotic summer. The fact that they embody the sacred feminine in their form.

My father has a massive fig tree. Each year it's a competition between me, the birds, the wasps and the butterflies for the harvest!

This is a beautiful late summer and autumn cake for when you have a glut of ripe fruit longing to be used. The original recipe from the River Café Easy cookbook was made with plums and almonds. I have also made it with frozen cherries and almonds, rhubarb and almonds, and peach and pecans. But our absolute favourite is this figgy version. For the nutty topping you can pick your own hazelnuts or cobnuts, or replace them with chopped almonds or pecans.

My version is gluten-free. It makes a delicious dessert accompanied by custard, cream or ice cream, or had at teatime (or breakfast!) with a cup of tea or coffee. It officially does keep well for a few days: good luck with that!

Lucy

Serves 8

For the fruit layer

500g (18oz) fruit (about 12 fresh figs)

1 orange – grated zest and juice

50g (2oz / ¼ cup) caster sugar

1 teaspoon vanilla extract

Pre-heat your oven to 170°C fan (180°C / 350°F / Gas mark 4).

Cut the fruit in half if using figs or plums (removing plum stones!). Place cut side down in a 23cm /

9in ovenproof dish or baking tin – this is what you will cook the cake in later, so make sure the sides are at least 5cm / 2in high. Add the orange rind, juice and vanilla. Put in the oven for 20 minutes. (If using cherries instead make sure they're stoned – you only need to put them in for 5 minutes).

For the cake

150g (5oz / 1½ sticks) butter

150g (5oz / ¾ cup) caster sugar

2 large eggs

150g (5oz / 1⅓ cup) ground almonds

35g (1½oz / 2½ tablespoons) cornflour/corn starch

1 teaspoon baking powder

Beat the butter and sugar together either by hand or in a food processor or with an electric whisk. Add in the eggs and whisk again. Add in the dry ingredients and whisk once more.

Pour this mixture on top of the fruit and return to the oven for another 30 minutes.

For the topping

30g (1½oz / 2 tablespoons) butter

30g (1½oz / 2 tablespoons) soft brown sugar

1 teaspoon vanilla extract

50g (2oz / ½ cup) chopped hazelnuts

Zest of one orange, grated

Pinch of sea salt flakes

In a small pan melt the butter and sugar. Stir through the remaining ingredients and remove it from the heat.

Pour evenly over the cake, lower the oven to 150°C fan (160°C / 310°F / Gas mark 2) and return the cake to the oven for 20 minutes more, keeping an eye on it so that the nuts don't burn.

Test with a skewer. If it is browning too fast and is still very wet inside cover with foil. It is cooked when brown on top and a skewer comes out clean.

No need for icing – this cake is delicious warm or cold.

Kitchen Witch Magic

Figs: connected to fire, as well as love and fertility.
Vanilla: for joy and good fortune.
Oranges: for sweetness, sunshine and fire.
Almonds: for abundance and fertility.

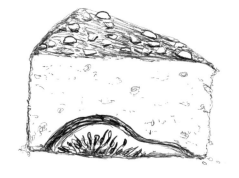

LATE AUTUMN

AUTUMN WREATH

This is the most abundant time of year for wreath making. There is so much beauty to choose from.

Red, yellow, brown and orange leaves. Maple, sycamore and beech have beautiful shapes and colours. Wild clematis, which I know as old man's beard, clusters of red berries – rose hips, rowan, hawthorn – or pink spindle berries, and silvery honesty pods. Unripe blackberries, juniper, sloes, spiky teasels, pinecones, crab apples, dried seed heads, spiky sea holly, moss, wheat and barley stems – green or golden, seeded grasses, gorse, acorns…

Either use a pre-made base, or shape some willow branches or ivy stems into a circle and bind with string or florists' wire. Weave in the greenery first, being sure to keep a visual balance, then add in berries and seed heads using thin florists' wire to attach.

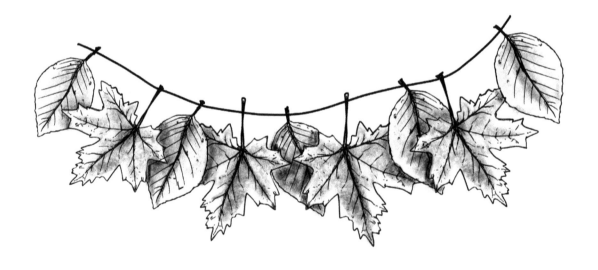

AUTUMN GARLANDS

Why not make a garland of crocheted or knitted leaves to hang above your mantelpiece. Or gather beautiful coloured leaves and thread them, dipping them in wax first if you want. Or thread rowan berries from the fairy tree onto strings for protection.

Hallowe'en

As a child, we used to try to catch doughnuts that hung from strings attached to a pulley with our hands behind our backs – the stickiness of the endeavour was part of the fun, and it felt like trying to bite the moon out of the sky – this was part of our Hallowe'en parties as children, alongside dooking for apples and reciting poetry.

Alice Tarbuck

At Hallowmas-Samhain I always leave a bowl of food by my garden gate for the ancestors. It feels important to not only honour my own beloved dead but also the collective ancestors who are held in the bones of the land.

Jacqueline

Forgotten Veg – Butternut Squash Soup

  CAN BE DAIRY FREE, VEGAN AND VEGETARIAN

I love the humble bumble of the butternut. It sits in my fridge for months, until there are no vegetables left in the house bar perhaps a shrivelled onion and a sprouting clove of garlic in the cupboard. This, and not a moment before, is when I relent and make butternut squash soup. And dear butternut never complains that he is always my last resort soup. But once made is always warming and delicious! This is also a fabulous soup for using up the flesh scooped from Halloween pumpkins.

Sarah

Makes 4 bowls or enjoy a bowl to yourself with plenty to freeze for later.

1 butternut squash or any eating pumpkin, halved longways, scoop out the seeds and remove stringy bits

1 onion

2 garlic cloves

1 litre (1¾ pints / 1 US quart) of stock of your choice – vegetable or chicken work best

2 teaspoons of oil – sesame is my favourite it mirrors the squashes nutty taste

Liberal salt and pepper

1 teaspoon smoked paprika

Optional: chilli fresh or dried for a spicy kick

Milk or cream for thinning/serving.

Preheat the oven to 190°C fan (200°C / 400°F / Gas mark 6).

Place the butternut squash on a baking tray or dish and drizzle each half with just enough olive oil to lightly coat the squash. Sprinkle it with salt, pepper and paprika.

Roast until it is tender and completely cooked through and brown at the edges, about 40 to 50 minutes. Set the squash aside to cool for a spell.

Meanwhile, in a large pan, warm 1 tablespoon oil over medium heat and soften the onion and garlic for a few minutes.

Scoop out all the flesh out with a spoon and discard the skin. Add the squash flesh to the pan.

Pour in the stock and bring the pan up to a gentle boil.

Then blend in the pan with a wand blender (or ladle into a regular blender and return to the pan for a final warm through).

If the mixture is very thick add some more water or stock, or a little milk or cream.

Pour into bowls, serve with a sprinkle of chilli flakes if desired.

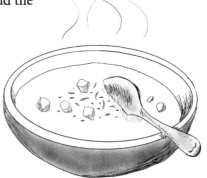

Kitchen Witch Magic

Butternut squash: all pumpkins and squashes symbolise abundance, fruitfulness, and good health.

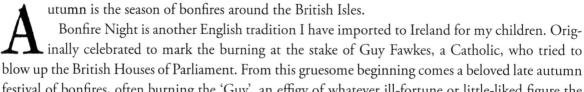

GATHERING – BONFIRE NIGHT

Remember, Remember! The Fifth of November,
The Gunpowder, treason and plot;
I know of no reason Why the Gunpowder treason
Should ever be forgot!

Autumn is the season of bonfires around the British Isles.

Bonfire Night is another English tradition I have imported to Ireland for my children. Originally celebrated to mark the burning at the stake of Guy Fawkes, a Catholic, who tried to blow up the British Houses of Parliament. From this gruesome beginning comes a beloved late autumn festival of bonfires, often burning the 'Guy', an effigy of whatever ill-fortune or little-liked figure the people want to be rid of that year as well as toffee apples and fireworks of all sorts.

In Ireland most fireworks are illegal – a hangover from years of sectarian battles – but we still have the bonfire and make and burn a Guy, we have sparklers and Chinese firecrackers, and gather friends and family to share mulled apple juice, hot chocolate and perhaps a bean stew with baked potatoes, consumed as we stand around the warmth of the dancing flames, wrapped in thick coats, scarves and hats. At last year's celebrations the night was mild enough and we sat out for hours watching an incredible display of shooting stars – the Leonid meteor shower – nature's very own fireworks!

Lucy

SMOKY BEAN STEW

  CAN BE MADE VEGAN, VEGETARIAN AND SUGAR FREE

I traditionally serve this for Bonfire Night celebrations as it is hearty, warming and filling, but it is great to take to potlucks too. It is a great store-cupboard dish to have up your sleeve when you have lots of friends over and suddenly have to feed a crowd at short notice during the autumn or winter. I make sure to keep plenty of tins of tomatoes and beans in the cupboard just in case! It is so easy to throw together a friend swore she didn't even notice me cooking it as I chatted. Her mind was blown when I served up dinner for 12!

I use chorizo in mine, but obviously omit it if you don't have it or don't eat pork. The smoked paprika is key to this dish, it is what is gives chorizo its distinctive colour and flavour and brings a smoky, savoury note which makes the stew so more-ish.

Serve with crusty bread, rice, couscous or baked potatoes (which you can put in the oven and then forget whilst you start on the stew). It works well as a burrito filling wrapped in tortillas with cheese, sour cream and fresh coriander (cilantro). It freezes well. Like most tomato-based stews it is even better the next day. It is also lovely served cold with chopped herbs, a sprinkle of feta or goats cheese and a drizzle of olive oil.

Lucy

Serves 10

3 x 450g (1lb) tins of chopped tomatoes

2 tablespoons oil – olive, sunflower or vegetable

2 tablespoons smoked paprika

2 tablespoons ground cumin

2 large onions chopped

A whole chilli – fresh or dried – chopped or left whole

3 x 450g (1lb) cans of beans – mixed beans, chickpeas (garbanzo), haricot, cannellini, kidney, black, black-eyed, butterbeans all work well, it's best with a mix of at least two.

5 cloves of garlic, minced. If you are in a rush/don't have fresh onions and garlic, use 2 tablespoons onion granules and 1 tablespoon garlic granules

Salt and pepper

Optional

Two sweet peppers (capsicums) (red, green or yellow) chopped into chunks

1 chorizo cut into cubes

1 tablespoon sugar or maple syrup

You will need the largest saucepan you have!

If you are using fresh onions, soften them in some oil in the pan over a medium heat for five minutes. Add the peppers and cook for another five minutes before adding the garlic and chorizo and frying for two more minutes, until the chorizo has released its oils. Add in the cumin and smoked paprika and fry for another minute.

Stir in the beans, chilli and salt and pepper. Pour over the chopped tomatoes and stir. Add the sugar if using. Add half a can of water. Cover and simmer on the stove top or in the oven for at least 20 minutes for the flavours to combine, but up to an hour on a low heat is fine.

Kitchen Witch Magic: Blessed beans

Beans have a long history of being associated with magic and other realms, as well use as amulets and talismans to offer protection. (We see this connection to magic carry into story like in the well-known fairy tale "Jack and the Beanstalk"). Multiple cultures associate eating or planting beans on certain days with good luck. In Europe it is best to plant beans on Good Friday. In areas of central America, newlyweds eat a bowl of beans for luck. On New Year's Day in areas of the southern United States and South America eating beans is considered to bring prosperity for the year.

Chickpeas (and butterbeans): comforting and soothing to the soul.
Haricot beans: strength and determination.
Kidney beans: represent wisdom, love, and healing. They are said to help to ward off evil spirits and protect against negative energy.
Black beans: creativity, wisdom and divination.
Black-eyed beans or peas: (and all beans) are considered connected to communication both between the material and the spirit realms and between people for example, for reconciliation.

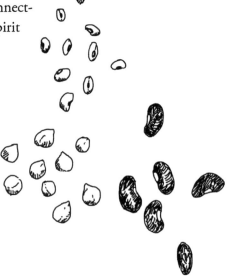

Ginger Syrup

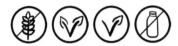

This delicious ginger syrup can be used to make a spectacular tea if mixed with hot water in around a 1:3 syrup to water ratio. It's also delicious with sparkling water and ice cubes, and with a tot of rum added, it warms the heart and belly.
Sarah

Makes 850ml (1½ pints / 4 cups)

450g (1lb / 4 cups) fresh ginger root – peeled and chopped

1 chilli

250ml/ (9fl oz / ¾ cup) honey

200g (7oz / 1 cup) brown sugar

450ml (16fl oz / 2 cups) water

Juice of 2 limes

Handful of coriander seeds

1 tablespoon black peppercorns

Add ginger to a large saucepan with chilli, honey, water, sugar, lime juice, coriander and peppercorns. Bring to the boil and simmer for 15 minutes. Leave to cool and infuse overnight. Strain through a cheesecloth or fine sieve and decant into a bottle. The syrup will last in the fridge for several weeks.

Kitchen Witch Magic

These are herbs and spices of heat: fiery and spicy as they may be, they support healing, soothing and peace.
Ginger: embodies this dual nature perfectly, it is both soothing for the stomach and connected to fiery, spicy energy. Fiery ginger, peppercorns and chilli can be empowering if consumed before spell or ritual work or working with the element of Fire.
Coriander seeds: to settle and soothe the stomach.
Honey and sugar: sweet and soothing.

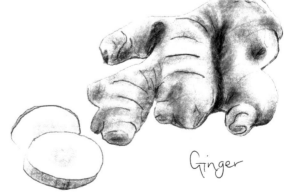

Ginger

SOUL CAKES

*There are many links between cakes and divination. In England
and Scotland, many young women would have baked special "dumb
cakes," either as part of a dumb supper or alone, to be eaten in silence
in order to invite a future husband to appear in her dreams.*

*Cakes have been used by people all over the world to honour their dead. The practice
of baking a soul cake or soul mass cake to commemorate and celebrate the dead for
Halloween, All Saints' Day and All Souls' Day in England dates back at least
to the medieval period. These small, round, spiced cakes were given out to children
and the poor who often went door to door to seek food and favour in return for
prayers and songs, in a practice called "souling." In this (along with the customs of
mumming and guising) we can see the roots of our modern custom of trick or treating.*

From *Kitchen Witch: Food, Folklore & Fairy Tale*

CATTERN CAKES

I love any of the spiced biscuits and cakes of the late autumn and winter that are made to be shared through trick or treating, wassailing, or carolling. Sharing is the greatest blessing, especially when those of us who have more than we need share with those who have less. It warms my cockles, and it's built into our winter traditions.

My favourite seasonal recipe is cattern cakes, which are a traditional English food of Catterntide, or St Catherine's Feast Day on 25th November. The almost-unchanged Tudor recipe includes cinnamon and caraway seeds added to a dough which is then rolled up and sliced with the hope that the resulting cakes will look like wheels.* Traditionally, they would be served with a 'hot pot' of rum, beer and eggs, but I usually stick to a nice cup of tea.

Catterntide is one of the doorways into the deep winter when we can make soul cake and harcake, or soulmass cake, for Hallowtide, or Samhain, and enjoy the community spirit of Stir-up Sunday†; such a warming, beautiful smelling time of year, and one built on sharing with the living and the dead across all worlds.

---

*   St Catherine was a Christian saint martyred in the early 4th century. She was tortured on a wheel and so she is remembered with Catherine Wheel fireworks at Bonfire Night and these wheel-shaped cakes.

†   A traditional day at the end of November (the last Sunday before the first Sunday of advent) in the UK when families gathered to make the Christmas cake and puddings, each stirring in wishes and luck.

There are some wonderful recipes and kitchen rituals connected to the saints. We think of them as cold and pious, but the pre-Reformation saints have warm and passionate hearts and bellies!

This recipe is adapted from one in *Cattern Cakes and Lace: a Calendar of Feasts* by Julia Jones and Barbara Deer. It can be easily tweaked for different dietary requirements. For example, my friend Jan Blencowe swaps the self-raising flour for paleo flour with two teaspoons of baking powder, substitutes flaked almonds for the ground almonds, and uses powdered stevia rather than caster sugar.

Jacqueline Durban

250g (9oz / 2¼ cups) self-raising flour, sieved. (Or add two teaspoons of baking powder to plain flour.)

Up to 2 teaspoons ground cinnamon (I do have a great love of cinnamon so you may want to start with less. I advise bold experimentation!)

50g (2oz / ⅓ cup) currants

50g (2oz / scant ½ cup) ground almonds

2 teaspoons caraway seeds

175g (6oz / ¾ cup) caster sugar

110g (4oz / 1 stick + 1 tablespoon) melted butter

1 medium egg, beaten

Extra sugar and cinnamon for sprinkling

Preheat your oven to 190°C fan (200°C / 400°F / Gas Mark 6).

Sieve the flour into a bowl and mix in all the other dried ingredients.

Add the melted butter and beaten egg and mix to form a soft dough. Add a tiny bit of warm water if needed.

Roll the dough out on a floured surface until you have a large rectangle (50cm x 25cm/20in x10in approximately).

Brush the rolled-out dough with water and then sprinkle with cinnamon (lots!) and sugar.

Gently roll lengthways, as though you are making a Swiss roll. It doesn't need to be too tight. Cut into 2cm wide slices and pop on a baking tray, leaving space in between to allow them to spread a little. Bake for about 10 minutes, or until golden and crispy on the top.

Bask in the loveliness as your house fills with the smell of spices and good things.

Remove your cakes from the oven and place on a wire rack to cool. You may see that they have a spiral pattern, which represents a Catherine Wheel. If not, don't worry, they will still taste delicious. You can sprinkle on some more caraway seeds at this point, and even more sugar and cinnamon if liked.

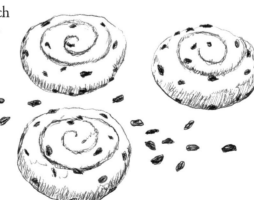

Once cool, they can be stored in an airtight container for up to seven days, but I can almost guarantee that they won't last that long. After all, Catterntide lasts for only one day!

Autumn Gratitude Simmer Pot

Autumn is a time to celebrate family, abundance and harvest, for appreciating all that we have and all that we've accomplished and utilizing the seasonal gifts we receive at this time of year. This blend is sweet, warm and bright with colours identical to autumn's leaves shining through.

Sarah Napoli

For this brew you will need:

Apples for love and protection.

Cinnamon for love and abundance.

Rosemary for cleansing and strength.

Sunflower for bringing forth happiness.

Cranberries for positivity and healing.

Bay leaves with each thing you're grateful for written on them.

Combine your ingredients. Stir clockwise and say:

I offer my gratitude and give thanks with this brew.
May the intentions I've set now flow on through.

Allow to simmer as long as desired and add water as needed.

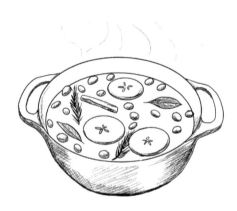

Hearthside Remembrance

We are all connected by a truth that we have lost people we love, to age or illness, to distance or conflict. This is a ritual to remember, allow yourself time to grieve a loss and create a space where you can feel your sorrows, angers and hurts.

Take your time to create a simmer pot – smell is so very tightly woven with memory, so you may want to follow the recipe above or create your own using smells that mean something to you, or that you are drawn to. I will always love the autumnal favourites: apple, orange, nutmeg, clove, ginger, cinnamon, vanilla, perhaps because I (Sarah) am an autumn baby, and because I find these scents soothing and heart-warming.

While the simmer pot gently steams, sit with a steaming brew, this might be drawn from the simmer pot if that is appropriate (not all simmer pot recipes are suitable for consumption), or your favourite herbal blend, coffee, mulled juice or wine (recipe p166), whatever you like.

You may wish to gather items to support your journey of remembrance – photos, gifts, a piece of jewellery or clothing. These can be placed before you, or around you.

Find a comfortable seat in your kitchen. Watch the rising plumes of steam around you – on the hob and in your hands.

Use your senses to ground you to this place for example:

Touch – warm cup, wooden table, any of your memorial items

Smell – the simmer pot, your hot drink

Sight – steam, flames, lights, your memorial items

Taste – your hot drink, a sweetness of honey or sugar added

Hearing – bubbling, crackling, any sounds of your home

When you feel ready speak aloud anything you are feeling about those you wish to remember (or write it down if that is more manageable). Feel your words, feel the emotions, let them rise and whirl like the steam around you.

Give yourself time to release – perhaps this takes the form of tears, or speaking aloud your thoughts, maybe you scream into a pillow or bang the ground. Sing, moan or chant. Perhaps you write down all you are feeling.

When you feel ready (and this is very personal, you may find yourself here for a few minutes or an hour, there is no time limit for feeling and releasing emotions, it is part of a much bigger journey of healing) take some deep breaths and finish your drink. Perhaps stretch your body if you wish and rise.

Thank your kitchen for holding space for you today as you turn off the simmer pot and put your memorial items somewhere safe, or perhaps add them to your altar space

Return to this space whenever you wish.

Blessing

May the nourishment of the Earth be yours,
May the clarity of light be yours,
May the fluency of the ocean be yours,
May the protection of the ancestors be yours.

"Blessing", John O'Donohue, from *Echoes of Memory*

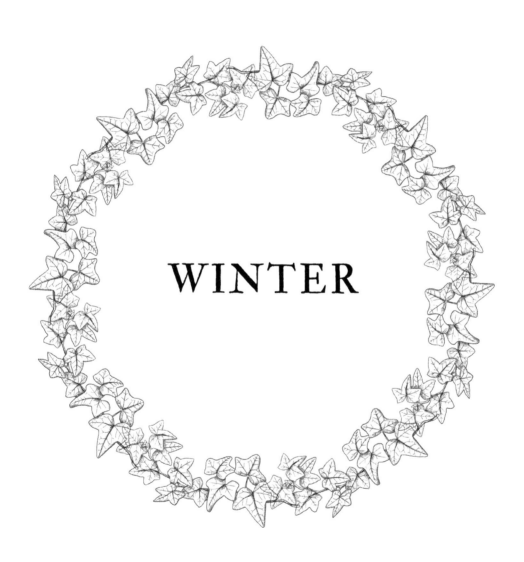

WINTER

Warming soups and broths, comforting casseroles, hot drinks that we wrap our hands around and savour, toast and crumpets with toppings melting onto plates and fingers, decadent cakes of warming fruits and spices, roasted winter vegetables that fill the house with earthy scents. It makes sense to eat delicious foods on the longest winter nights, for we often need a little extra comfort and warmth in the dark. Much of the hedgerow and its residents are sleeping. Much is bare and brown. Ivy berries ripen and are gobbled up by starlings, thrushes, and wood pigeons, and perhaps the last of the holly berries, rosehips, and sloes. The nights are long and dark. There may be snow and ice. But after the midwinter solstice, each day lengthens just a little. And come January, we may see the first snowdrops reaching through the earth. This flower is also known in England by a variety of folk names 'Candlemas bells', 'February fair maids' and 'snow piercers' (like the French name for the flowers *perce-neige*).

Winter is a time of hibernation, celebrations of feasting, light, hope and togetherness during the darkest of days. When light and warmth in the season are scarce, how blessed we are to be able to create our own! It is easy (and understandable) to become a little cynical around the pressures and mindless consumerism of the festive season. But this can be a time to mindfully create what you wish. Longing for time to rest with books on dark evenings? This is what the wonderful Icelandic tradition of the 'Yule book flood' is all about. Embrace the Scandinavian practice of *hygge* by focusing on all the ways you can conjure cosyness. Enjoy bringing loved ones together with favourite foods? Make time for these things! You may wish to leave the hustle of the high street for early morning walks in frosted woodlands, or swap buying gifts for baking them instead. For centuries, the light and warmth of revelries has always been more about the people, laughter, comfort, charity and companionship, or time for reflection and meditation, than gifts. So focus on creating memories, laughter, comfort, offering your time to those in need of company. No money is needed for these foundations of the season and the most precious rituals do not involve consumerism, despite what clever marketing would have us believe.

Winter festivals include: Thanksgiving, Candlemas, Diwali (Festival of Lights), St Lucia's Day, Kwanzaa, Winter Solstice, Yule, Christmas Eve and Day, St Stephen's or Boxing Day, Hogmanay, New Year's Eve and Day, Women's Little Christmas and Epiphany and Burns Night.

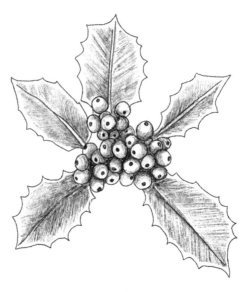

KITCHEN TABLE CHARMS

Decorate with evergreens, a timeless tradition – look for ivy, fir, bay, pine to make boughs over doorframes, mantles, and windows. Whatever size of home you have and however small your budget you can fill a jar with some bare winter branches and hang with twinkling baubles, fairy lights, threaded winter berries, crocheted snowflakes or silver foil origami stars.

New Year – In Scotland the 'first footing' is the first visitor after midnight on New Year's Eve, and lore dictates they should come bearing gifts symbolising ingredients for a prosperous year such as warmth, food, money, and good cheer (these may be symbolised with offerings of coal, bread, coins and whisky). You may wish to place symbolic items on your kitchen table such as a freshly baked cake or cookies for a year of sweetness and hospitality, or a candle for a year of light and warmth. Or even gather your nearest and dearest for the New Year's Day meal in an invocation of a year full of such gatherings.

SEASONAL MEDITATION: WINTER

Close your eyes and relax as we settle and breathe.

We find ourselves within our mind's eye on a walk on a winter's morning – a milky haze hangs heavy over valleys and fields, trees have shed their leaves and frost sparkles on dawn grasses. You spot evergreen plants, the red berries of holly and white of mistletoe. Looking closer you see amongst the frosted hedgerows, the glow of crimson rosehips and darkest purple sloes.

You move amongst trees into woodland and spot sweet chestnuts, their spiny casings on the ground amongst the leaves of the winter woodland floor. You gather just a few as a treat and take them home to your cosy and warm house.

Walking inside you discard your winter coat and scarf and gloves and sit before a crackling fire, taking a seat upon soft blankets. You roast the chestnuts over the open fire and eat them warm.

You feel that warmth in your belly. In the past, the winter dark would have held some trepidation and anxiety: a multitude of unknowns could leave people starving and freezing. You feel grateful that you will not have such worries but hold respect for the challenges of getting up in the dark, inclement weather, and the low light levels. It is a time to really look after yourself. In these dark nights, with an energy of mindfulness, and the dormant season of the earth, we have a chance to pause and reflect.

What paths and journeys have brought you here to this point? What gifts have you been blessed with over the year and festive season? Have you taken time to be truly grateful for the roof above your head and food on your plate? What are your wishes for the year ahead?

You pause in this place, before the crackling fire, feasting on nature's bounty.

What does the dark of winter bring up for you? Where can you shine light in the darkness? What could you let fall away like the dry winter leaves from a tree? How might you rest and create cosiness in celebration of the long dark nights?

If you would like to journal with these questions, feel free to take time after your meditation to write.

EARLY WINTER

Winter Wreath

Although the plant world seems to be sleeping in midwinter, there are still many leaves, berries and even flowers to be found – hydrangea, eucalyptus, fir, spruce, holly, ivy, moss, rosemary, rosehips, hawthorn and holly berries, pine and alder cones, teasels and dried allium or Agapanthus heads (these look fabulous sprayed gold, silver or fake-snow covered).

Either use a pre-made base, or shape some willow branches or ivy stems into a circle and bind. Weave in the greenery first, being sure to keep a visual balance, then add in your decorations using thin florists' wire to attach. There are many winter fruits and spices which can be added to your wreath to add colour, texture and scent:

- ☾ cranberries threaded onto wire

- ☾ popcorn strings

- ☾ oranges, lemons, kumquats or limes – these can be cut into slices or left whole and slashed down the sides and dried overnight in a very low oven, or studded with cloves

- ☾ dried apple slices

- ☾ physalis (golden Chinese gooseberries in their papery brown cases)

- ☾ pink spindle berries

- ☾ threaded dried rowan berries

- ☾ crab apples

- ☾ red chillies

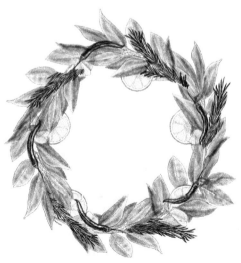

As well, of course, as all manner of magical tinsel, glitter, sparkle, snow spray, artificial flowers, Christmas baubles and bells.

Why not make an edible winter herbal wreath from rosemary, bay leaves and chillies? It is both a beautiful decoration and a great excuse to prune back the old year's growth on your evergreen herb bushes. You can keep this in the kitchen until well into the spring – using up the dried bay leaves and chillies, rather than having to brave the wet and cold when making a winter stock or stew. These also make beautiful and useful gifts for family and friends.

Winter Garlands

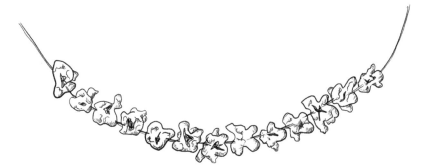

December is traditionally a time for adorning the house, with a Christmas tree, advent wreath and evergreens. There can be lots of pressure to purchase decorations. We have always erred on the side of homemade. Some lovely edible ways of decorating your home, which can be done with children or sat around a table with friends, include gingerbread decorations, strings of popcorn and cranberries! Taking a needle and thread you can make popcorn strings as a homemade tree decoration which looks a little like snow. Or thread fresh cranberries onto thin flexible wire and make into hoops or heart shapes to hang on your wreath or tree.

If you have needle skills why not make crochet stars or snowflakes and either thread them onto a long cord as a garland to hang over your mantelpiece or make them on individual loops to hang on bare branches in a vase or onto a Christmas tree.

A simple salt dough made of water, flour and salt can be rolled out and cut into Christmassy shapes, baked in a low oven until hard and then decorated with poster or acrylic paints, and varnished with a simple mix of PVA glue and water. These inexpensive homemade decorations will last for years.

Creating Christmas

This is the time of Christmas parties, traditionally times of excess and inebriation. Our women's group created a different sort of Christmas party that didn't rely on alcohol to lift the spirits. Each year we found a couple of simple craft projects that our mixed-ability group was able to do – threading festive coloured buttons onto wire to make heart-shaped decorations, binding twigs to make stars, salt dough decorations, twigs tied to make tiny Christmas trees – check out my Pinterest boards for an array of ideas.* We would each bring a festive treat to eat or drink, and would sing carols together at the end. In later years we have gathered for a meal and then walked a winter solstice spiral (from the Steiner Waldorf tradition) – usually made of ivy and evergreens laid out on the floor, lit with nightlight candles in pots. During covid times when we couldn't gather indoors, we met at the local beach and drew a spiral in the sand, illuminated with storm lamps.

* Pinterest.com/dreamingaloudnt

Gathering together with a few dear friends can bring magic to a crazy time – with a gentle focus on light, creativity, rest, and feasting together on healing spices and foods…

Lucy

My favourite season is usually the one that we are travelling through at the time but, if I had to choose one, it would be winter. I find midwinter so deep with meaning and so rich with tradition. I love the feeling of snuggling up to tell stories around a fire, real or metaphorical, with a hot bowl of soup and spiced ale. One of my favourite quotes comes from Dickens: 'I will honour Christmas in my heart, and try to keep it all year.'

Jacqueline Durban

MULLED DRINKS

Star Anise

Glühwine or mulled wine is indelibly linked to the cold season here in Northern Europe. As a non-red wine drinker, my favourite winter drink is a mulled apple juice. This is our go to cold-season drink, from Christmas parties to bonfire nights – it is loved by children and adults alike. The mulling spices can also be used in red wine. And if some of your guests want to add a tipple to stave off the cold, it's delicious with a dash of brandy – apple or apricot are good – or whisky. Both the spices and the temperature are warming.

You can also bag up the sugar and spice mix and gift it with a gift tag of instructions – but you'll need to dry the orange in a slow oven overnight or leave it out.

Lucy

1 cinnamon stick

1 orange sliced

8 cloves

5 cardamom pods

1 star anise

50g (2oz / 3 tablespoons) caster sugar (to taste)

1 litre (1¾ pints / 1 quart) cloudy apple juice (not from concentrate)/apple cider/ pomegranate juice/red wine

Put all ingredients in a pan and cover. Warm gently on a hob without boiling for at least 15 minutes, up to an hour to infuse. Taste and adjust sweetness as needed. Ladle into mugs – adding a dash of spirits at this point (if using) to preserve the alcohol.

Kitchen Witch Magic

Star anise: has a beautiful star shape and strong aniseed flavour. It is often used for purification and cleansing, and is burned in temples and sacred spaces in Japan.

Cinnamon: for warming, connected to sun and fire.

Cloves: intense, aromatic, and spiky, cloves are the dried flower buds of the clove tree and used in folk medicine for salves and balms to offer pain relief from toothache, headache, and joint pain. The name "clove" derives from the Latin *clavus,* meaning nail. Both cloves and nails (like the ones often found in warding witch bottles) are strongly connected with protection and driving away negative energy. Perfect for dark winter nights when the shadows fall and moods can drop.

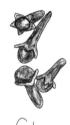

Cloves

Sarah – A new ritual my partner and I have begun in our new home is to light our firepit on Christmas Eve with a mug of well-spiced mulled wine.

IMMUNI-TEA

This is a low sugar version of mulled apple juice that I developed for my winter mornings, as someone who doesn't drink tea or coffee. It's also great after chilly winter walks, or being caught in the rain, with lots of immune boosting ingredients to avert shivers and sneezes. It's also faster than the mulled apple juice in the previous recipe, as quick as a cuppa to make.

Lucy

100ml (4fl oz / ½ cup) cloudy apple juice (not from concentrate)

100ml (4fl oz / ½ cup) boiling water

Half a cinnamon stick

Grated fresh ginger to taste (½–1 teaspoon)

10 drops echinacea tincture (or ½ teaspoon of dried root)

Juice of ¼–½ a lemon (to taste)

Optional if you have them/if you like the taste/want added sweetness/need more immune boosting power

1 teaspoon manuka honey

1 teaspoon elderberry syrup

Put all ingredients straight in your cup, stir. Hold the cup in your chilly hands, breathe in the steam, then drink.

Cinnamon

Kitchen Witch Magic

Manuka Honey: all honey is powerful for healing, but manuka is the 'bee knees' (snigger!) as the manuka flowers that the bees feed from to create this special honey have their own unique healing properties. Because of its specialness manuka honey is expensive, if it's not practical to invest in manuka honey – then heather or eucalyptus honey are also wonderful. All source flowers add their own properties to the honey (a takeaway point here being brands that use responsibly sourced honey will know from which plants and areas their bees have been feeding – large nameless supermarket brands may well not and may in fact feed their bees on sugar syrup).

Echinacea: for healing and protection.

Propolis: one of nature's most magical gifts in my opinion when it comes to the treatment of sore throats, colds, infections and even small cuts. It is a natural resin-like product made by bees and so powerful that a small bottle of pure propolis can see a family of four through several years of illnesses and small accidents.

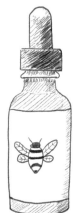

You can dilute a few drops of propolis in a glass of water, or simply put some on a teaspoon and swallow it. It will coat your swollen tonsils as you do so, soothing and instantly protecting. It does the same for small cuts; the combination of anti-bacterial properties to fight infection and the wax-like resin to seal small wounds is simply miraculous. As with all by products from bees, it is also a great immune booster.

Indra Roelants

CRANBERRIES

Jacqueline Durban

In the winter dark of 2021 I fell deeply in love with cranberries. They are so pleasingly firm and plump, and that beautiful deep red colour, enough to warm the dullest of winter days. I especially enjoyed making them into garlands for our kitchen and garden trees.

But imagine my delight when I was told that they grow in bogs and fens! Truly, they are a being of the edge places. Most of the berries we see in our supermarkets in Europe are cultivated in the US, Canada and Chile in managed bogs and exported into Europe. It's possible to find the most wonderful images of expanses of water whose almost entire surface is awash with cranberries. It really is the most surreal sight.

Cranberries grow on long, low-lying evergreen vines that, undamaged, can survive for centuries. When growing in acidic, nutrient-poor bogs, the plant's mycorrhizae help it to obtain nutrients. Their name comes from the similarity of their pink flowers to the head, neck, and beak of a crane, hence crane-berry/cranberry. In the US, they are sometimes known as bearberries, and the traditional English name for the plant is fenberry, a smaller berried native species that grows in the fens and marshes of

England. In Wales they are *llygaeron* and *ceiros-y-waun,* in Scotland, *mùileag,* and in Ireland, *mónóg,* meaning 'peat berry'.

Cranberries have been gathered in Europe for millennia. They have been found in a fermented mead buried with a young woman who died sometime between 1500 and 1300 BCE in Egtved, Denmark. An Irish monastic manuscript on wound care, dating to 1352 CE, recommends the seeds in a drink for those with inflamed wounds. In 1597, Gerard spoke of gathering the wild berries he called 'marrish whortes' or 'fenne-berries' near Cheshire and Staffordshire, noting that, "they take away the heate of the burning agues"; deeply useful as the ague, or marsh malaria, was prevalent where cranberries grew, having been brought here from Africa and the Middle East by Roman soldiers. One of my favourite saints, Pega of the Fens, was cast out when her brother, Guthlac, who considered denial of the body a spiritual act, thought that the Devil had visited him in the shape of his sister and tempted him to eat a crust of bread before sunset. It's likely that he was suffering from ague and was experiencing hallucinations, but their story is also a reminder that kitchen witchery is about rejoicing in our bodies' need for nutrition and delicious delights, rather than miserable self-denial.

The Gentleman's Magazine and Historical Chronicle of December 1829, tells us that, prior to the Enclosures and the draining of the fens, between 2–4,000 pecks (16 pints = 1 peck) of cranberries might be collected in a year, being sold for five shillings per peck. After the drainage of the fens, far fewer plants survived and so sold for 30–50 shillings per peck. This is how, and why, foods become luxury items, and the food of the rich. Land justice is food justice.

The legendary epic of Finland, the *Kalevala,* recounts the tale of Marjatta, a virgin who, whilst wandering in the forests, hears the singing of the cranberry, which begs her to eat him. After doing so she becomes pregnant and is shunned by her family who refuse to believe her story. Later, she gives birth to her son in a stable in a forest. No wonder that cranberries are so deeply woven into Christmastide! Writer, Shirley Twofeathers goes further, suggesting adding a bowl of cranberries to our Hallowmas altar to show thanks to the supernatural powers of the bog where our ancestors once made offerings, and including cranberries into a small protective wreath to hang over our doorways during the long winter dark.

In the British Isles, cranberries are firmly a food of Christmas, to be added to cakes and pies and made into cranberry jelly, and so quickly disappear from our shops once the festivities are over. I look forward to their return. Truly, they hold in their bittersweet hearts an alternative map of the world: one where the Christmas story unfolds in a Finnish forest and a peck of wild cranberries sustains the poor. One day perhaps, in defiance of the Enclosures and the drainage of the fens, like Marjatta, I will hear their wild song.*

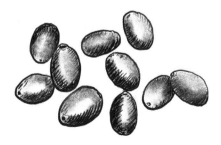

---

*   See Bibliography for references.

CRANBERRY CHRISTMAS CAKE

I am not one for old fashioned fruit cakes – although I love all the customs around them and have memories of stirring the Christmas Cake on Stir Up Sunday in late November with my mother, and the ritual of giving it a weekly drink of brandy until the day came to ice it. I always wished the flavour lived up to the fun of the ritual and the beauty of the snowy white icing adorned with carefully cut out fondant holly leaves and berries. But the truth is I really don't like dark raisiny fruit cakes and can't stand marzipan.

In Ireland we have something called a White Christmas Cake that I like more than the dark currant and raisin packed traditional varieties. This recipe came via my dear friend and doll-maker extraordinaire, Laura Whalen.

I have adapted it to be gluten-free and with extra fruity goodness. The sour bursts of crimson cranberries make it refreshing and festive looking and the crystallised ginger is magically zingy. If you want to make it and can't get your hands on fresh cranberries they can be replaced with fresh or frozen raspberries or cherries.

This is a low rise, moist cake which keeps well – though in our house it rarely lasts a day! Unlike a traditional Christmas cake it will not be there waiting for when guests call unexpectedly into early January, but is super-fast to mix up…and fills the kitchen with a beautiful festive smell of orange, cranberry, cardamom, toasty nuts and ginger.

If you need it to be nut-free replace the ground almonds and rice flour/cornflour mix with ½ cup (60g / 2oz) plain flour and omit the pecans.

Lucy

1 egg

110ml (4fl oz / ½ cup) orange juice – taken from the orange you zest (topping it up with juice from a carton is fine)

3 tablespoons vegetable oil

75g (3oz / ⅓ cup) caster sugar

2 teaspoons baking powder

1 teaspoon ground cardamom

50g (2oz / ½ cup) ground almonds

½ teaspoon salt

30g (1oz / ¼ cup) made up of half cornflour (cornstarch) and half rice flour/standard gluten-free flour

150g (5oz / 1 cup) fresh cranberries

Grated zest of one orange

4 tablespoons crystallised ginger – chopped

30g (1oz / ¼ cup) chopped pecans

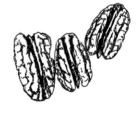

1 medium (500g / 1lb) loaf tin
Preheat the oven to 170°C fan (180°C / 350°F / Gas mark 4)

In a jug whisk the egg, oil and orange juice together until combined.

In a bowl stir together the sugar, baking powder, ground cardamom, ground almonds, cornflour and rice flour, make a well in the centre.

Tip the wet ingredients into the dry. Stir to combine. Add in the fruit, orange zest, ginger and pecans.

Pour the batter (don't panic, it is VERY wet!) into a lined standard loaf tin. Bake for 35–40 mins. Test with a skewer after 30 minutes. If it is browning too fast and is still very wet inside cover with foil. It is cooked when brown on top and a skewer comes out clean.

No need for icing – this is delicious warm or cold with a cup of tea.

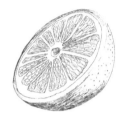

Kitchen Witch Magic

Pecans: abundance and prosperity.
Oranges: uplifting and a good source of vitamin C.
Cardamom: soothes and settles the stomach and warms us inside.
Ginger: warmth, raising energy and good health, soothes headaches and settles the stomach.

CRANBERRY MINCEMEAT

Mince pies are the traditional Christmas treat in the British Isles, served for centuries, most people now buy them. They are easy enough to make and fill your kitchen with the most Christmassy scents. A long way back they would have contained meat – hence the name! More recently they contained just suet, a hard animal fat which when melted makes an unctuous rich filling. These contain no suet and so are perfect for vegetarians and vegans! The cranberries and apples help to thicken the spiced raisin filling.

Make your own buttery shortcrust pastry or use store-bought. Cut it into rounds, popping them into a 12-hole baking tray, fill each with a dollop of mincemeat and top with a lid – or a small pastry star. Bake for 10 minutes. Serve warm or cold, by themselves of with brandy butter, whipped cream or ice cream.

Alternatively add an extra peeled, cored apple to the mix, spread over a sheet of puff pastry and roll into a log. Glaze with some milk, sprinkle with demerara sugar and bake for 30–40 minutes to make a beautiful warming winter strudel to feed a whole table.

Or spoon onto the bottom of a cake tin and then continue with the recipe for fig and hazelnut cake.

Lucy

1 bag of fresh cranberries (about 250g / 9oz / 2¾ cups)

450g (1lb) cooking apples

1 teaspoon each ground cinnamon and mixed spice

100g (4oz / ⅔ cup) chopped mixed peel (candied citrus peel)

100g (4oz / ⅔ cup) sultanas

100g (4oz / ⅔ cup) raisins

50g (2oz / ½ cup) flaked almonds, crushed in your hand

100ml (4fl oz / ½ cup) port

120g (4½oz / 1¼ cup) soft brown sugar

Juice of 1 orange

Bubble it all over a medium heat, stirring to prevent it sticking, until all the cranberries have exploded and it's syrupy – about 15 minutes. Test for sweetness. Take off the heat and add…

A generous slosh of brandy/Grand Marnier

1 teaspoon vanilla extract

Keep in a jar in the fridge and use to fill mince pies.

Kitchen Witch Magic

Cranberries: high in antioxidants, cranberries can be symbolic of cleansing and rejuvenation. They also symbolise abundance, courage, action. Popular for harvest feasts, especially in America where they grow, and English roast dinners during autumn and winter.

Celebrations

Mince pies have had many names on their journey from their first incarnations in medieval times, one such name was 'wayfarers' pies' – as they were given to travellers to warm their bellies on long winter nights. We strongly encourage celebrating the spirit of Yuletide by making a batch this winter and offering to a homeless shelter or charity. They would also make the perfect gift for anyone who is about to embark on a new path or challenge. The warmth from the spices is very fine, and baking these pies as gifts, showing someone you care is very powerful heart-warming magic as well.

Gingerbread

A traditional European Christmas treat…to be cut out as hearts, people, stars, snowflakes…or dinosaurs in our house on occasion! I love the symbolic magic of choosing the cutters. At Halloween we make them to give to our neighbours when our children trick or treat. The adults are always delighted to get an unexpected something. Gingerbread people are decorated with white strips of icing to make mummies and circles are squashed slightly and a small stem added to make pumpkins, which we give Jack O'Lantern faces with icing once cooked. At Christmas they can be hung on the tree, eaten at a party or gifted. This quantity is enough for a medium gingerbread house, which can be stuck together with hot toffee or royal icing and decorate with lots of sweeties – do mind your fingers if you use hot toffee as glue. Royal icing is a better choice if there are kids involved or you, like me, are accident-prone.

This is a super simple one pot recipe perfect for novice bakers of all ages. The biscuits are easy – building a gingerbread house that stays up and looks good…not so much!

Lucy

100g (3½oz / 1 stick) butter

50g (2oz / ¼ cup) white sugar

50g (2oz / ¼ cup) soft brown sugar

200g (7oz / ⅔ cup) golden syrup (or ⅓ cup corn syrup and ⅓ cup molasses)

400g (14oz / 2 cups) plain flour

1 tablespoon baking powder

2 teaspoon ground ginger

1 teaspoon ground cinnamon

1 teaspoon vanilla extract

Preheat the oven to 170°C fan (180°C / 350°F / Gas mark 4)

First make the gingerbread. Melt the sugars, syrup and butter gently in a large pan. Remove from the heat. Stir in the flour and spices. Stir until combined.

Pour onto a sheet of baking paper. Roll out to about ½cm / ¼in thick. Using cutters cut out into shapes.

Bake for 10–15 minutes, keep a careful eye on them so they don't go too dark around the edges. Cool on a wire rack before icing. Un-iced they keep well for a couple of weeks in an airtight tin and are crisp. Iced they keep fine but are soft.

Kitchen Witch Magic

Golden syrup: a golden elixir made from sugar cane grown in the sun, perfect for bringing a warmth, light and comforting energy to foods.

WINTER SOLSTICE MEAD

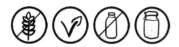

Mead is a fermented raw honey beverage that has been made for thousands of years in Europe as well as parts of Asia and Africa. There's something about this most ancient of drinks that our ancestors knew well that thrills me. What better brew to offer up to them in ceremony and ritual, to give thanks to the land and the people gone before us?

Mead was an integral part of a king's coronation ceremony in ancient and medieval Ireland, and *Medb* – the old Celtic word for mead – was also the name of the legendary queen of Connacht in Irish mythology.

The oldest drink found by archaeologists in pottery was of mead with grapes, rice and hawthorn. I was so happy to read this because my most successful meads seem to be the ones which I call 'bastardised' or rather a hybrid between a fruit alcohol and a honey alcohol.

You can make mead with modern brewing techniques, by boiling the honey with water and cooling rapidly and then adding a specially bought commercial yeast strain, such as that used to make champagne. This method will give you a consistent predictable outcome… but where's the fun in that?

I don't add commercial brewing yeast to my meads, preferring instead to continue the ancient brewing tradition of harnessing the already present wild yeasts that are just waiting to do their thing. Wild yeast will lead to a more complex flavour and it's safe to say that no mead will ever be the same as the next one! The honey itself contains the very yeasts needed to ferment it. All we have to do is activate them by adding water. Yeasts developed in factories I guess are designed to give consistent results but to me that defeats the whole excitement of fermentation and the variations that unfold. Who are we to say which kind of yeast 'should' prevail when we know that there is a far greater wisdom out there that we as humans can tap into if we just let everything be!

I'm in the habit of making small brews of mead – I call these 'mini meads' (an Austin Powers reference which totally dates me!) – primarily because they're much easier to tend to. I don't need huge amounts, and it makes it seem far more precious. Good local raw honey is something to be mindful of, no drop will go to waste. We don't need huge amounts of something for it to be highly beneficial and powerful. I try to make these on or for the eight festivals throughout the year.

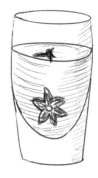

I'm learning to give a generous drop to the ancestors first before the living humans. This small acknowledgement and ritual expression of gratitude to those who have gone before us can make a profound change in one's life.

1.5 litre (3 pint / 1½ quart) clip top (Kilner) jar

1 x 450g (1lb) jar of local raw honey (that hasn't been heated over 43°C / 110°F)

500g (1lb) fruit – made up of hawthorn berries, elderberries (dried), blackberries (frozen)

Water to top up

Put all ingredients into the Kilner jar and stir well. Fasten the lid and leave to brew on a countertop in a warm place in your kitchen. For the first couple of days it's a good idea to stir it twice a day if you can.

Once bubbles of carbon dioxide start appearing, make sure the lid is secure and continue to allow it to ferment in a warm place for about 3 weeks.

This can be served neat for celebrations or diluted as a great warming winter drink, put a shot of this in a mug with a teaspoon of honey and top up with hot water.

Penny Allen

Winter Solstice Simmer Pot

In the dead of winter, the solstice is a welcome reminder of the sun's return. We have reached the longest night of the year meaning the days are officially getting longer and warmer. This brew holds a refreshingly crisp and spiced scent and is intended to connect you to this natural shift by utilizing ingredients associated with this time of year.

For this brew you will need:

Cranberries for abundance.

Rosemary for protection.

Oranges to honour the sun and positivity.

Cedar, a Yule correspondence associated with longevity.

Hypericum berries for good tidings.

Cinnamon for love.

Cloves for home protection.

Allspice for luck and healing.

Combine your ingredients. Stir clockwise and say:

We welcome the warmth and return of the sun.
Intentions now set, coming forth one by one.

Allow to simmer as long as desired and add water as needed.

Sarah Napoli

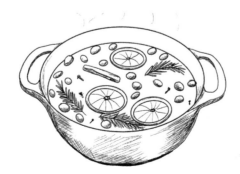

Candle Magic – Finding a Light in the Dark

Whatever our beliefs, we instinctively light candles to create an intimate, romantic or magical feeling in a room. The flicker of candlelight and dimmer light helps us to feel calm and connected.

Lighting candles is a simple and powerful way of creating a personal connection to the light during the dark of winter. It also connects us with our ancestors who would have lit their nights and winters with the flickering light of fire, lamp and candle.

Candle magic is an ancient form of sympathetic magic. Candles are used in rituals to represent people, things, and emotions. Casting a spell focuses one's intent to influence the desired outcome represented by the candle. In addition, one may use pyromancy: divination through gazing upon the flames of your candle. And if you have a fireplace, you can gaze into these flames too. Hold a question or guidance you are seeking in your mind, see what comes to mind or what images dance in the flames. Burning petitions or offerings for spellwork can also be useful and beautiful.

Coloured candles are used for their symbolic correspondences. The correspondences below are drawn from various alchemical and astrological resources, which may vary depending on your school of thought and own intuition.

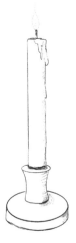

- ☾ Red signifies courage, health and passion.
- ☾ Pink signifies friendship and love.
- ☾ Purple signifies power, wisdom, spirituality and meditation.
- ☾ Orange signifies encouragement, attraction and adaptability.
- ☾ Gold and yellow signify success, the sun's energy and abundance.
- ☾ Blue signifies health, knowledge and patience.
- ☾ Green signifies fertility and abundance.
- ☾ Black signifies healing and transformation.
- ☾ White signifies truth, protection and peace.
- ☾ Brown is related to the Earth goddesses, elementals and animals.
- ☾ Silver signifies intuition and lunar connections.

You may wish to anoint the candle with essential oil connected to symbolic or healing qualities. If your goal is to draw something toward you, anoint from the ends of the candle inwards to the middle. To repel something, rub from the centre to the ends. You may also want to carve words, runes or symbols into the wax. Take your time to meditate or set intentions with your candle as you light it.

May you always find your own light in the dark.

LATE WINTER

FIRE CIDER IMMUNE BOOSTER

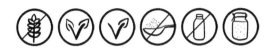

Fire cider is a folk remedy consisting of warming and stimulating ingredients soaked in apple cider vinegar. Herbal vinegar tonics, such as Four Thieves Vinegar, have been crafted amongst herbalists for many years, but the fire cider we know today originally got its name from American herbalist Rosemary Gladstar. While you will find many recipes for fire cider that differ from Gladstar's original, the intention for an immune boosting brew still stands. Because fire cider holds anti-inflammatory, antibacterial, antiviral, antimicrobial, and antifungal properties it is used to help combat many common ailments such as colds, flus, seasonal illnesses and allergies. It is also a stimulant for the digestive system.

Many of the ingredients you will see used here have their own magical associations as well, including, but not limited to: protection, cleansing and banishing of negative energy. Magical correspondences are just a little something extra I like to think about when crafting an herbal remedy such as this.

If you find yourself unable to locate one or two of these ingredients, don't fret, they may be replaced by another immune boosting ingredient or simply left out. Some alternatives for the ingredients listed here could be: oranges, cayenne peppers or star anise.

1 litre (1¾ pint / 1 quart) mason or Kilner jar

600–700ml (1–1½ pints / 3–4 cups) of apple cider vinegar with "The Mother"

1 white onion cubed

2 jalapeño chillies halved

50g (2oz / ⅓ cup) grated horseradish root

50g (2oz / ⅓ cup) grated ginger root

Parchment (baking) paper

1 lemon sliced

3 pieces of fresh turmeric peeled and diced

6–10 cloves of garlic

2 sprigs of rosemary (1 tablespoon dried)

1 tablespoon peppercorns

1 tablespoon dried thyme

1 cinnamon stick

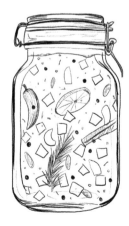

Combine your ingredients leaving about 3–5cm (1–2in) from the top of your jar. Top it off with the apple cider vinegar and cover with parchment paper before capping. Allow to sit for 4–6 weeks. You may strain your ingredients or blend everything together and add honey to taste. Store for up to 12 months in a cool dark cupboard. Take as a shot or mix with water once a day to utilize its immune boosting properties. Fire cider may also be used in cooking as you would use any other vinegar.

Kitchen Witch Magic

Ginger, chillies and horseradish: bring a fiery flavour.
Garlic and onions: for their immune boosting abilities.
Turmeric: for its anti-inflammatory properties and golden fiery colour.

    Sarah Napoli

KHICHDI – FOOD THAT FEELS LIKE A HUG

   VEGAN AND DAIRY FREE IF YOU USE NON-DAIRY SPREAD

The magical quality of food is the ability to make you feel like you are receiving a hug even without the arms of a loved one around you. It's the aroma that transports you into a warm cocoon of familiarity and safety. The texture that makes you feel soothed as it travels through your mouth. For me the dish that makes me feel this way is khichdi.

Khichdi is the inspiration for the Anglo-Indian dish kedgeree. In its simplest essence khichdi is a dish consisting of lentils and rice. My association goes all the way to being weaned on it as my first solid food. It is the Indian comfort food equivalent to chicken soup, the dish that is cooked when mourning the loss of someone. My favourite time to eat khichdi is on rainy days when I have nothing to eat or when I am missing the comforts of home. The additions of red onions or poppadom gives the dish a crunch if like me you enjoy different textures in your meal.

Each region of India and household has its own variation to this soul-touching food. My variation is a version adopted from my mum and adds the flare of my paternal family's need for spice. In traditional Indian cooking all ingredients are eyeballed because recipes are passed down orally instead of written down. But this the basic recipe to make your own.

    Khyati Patel

Serves 2

50g (2oz) whole moong beans

30g (1oz) split yellow moong dal lentils

70g (3oz) rice

450ml (16fl oz) water (plus more to loosen the consistency)

1 teaspoon asafoetida

1 teaspoon fenugreek seeds

1 teaspoon salt

1 teaspoon turmeric

1 teaspoon ground black pepper

1 tablespoon ghee (or butter and oil mixed or non-dairy alternative)

Soak the beans and lentils together and the rice separately in tap water for 30 minutes. Once soaked, rinse the ingredients until the water runs clear.

Bring 450ml of water to a boil in a lidded saucepan and add the beans and lentils along with the asafoetida, fenugreek seeds, turmeric, salt, pepper, and ghee. Bring back to the boil then simmer for 15 minutes.

Once the beans are slightly soft add the rice along with more water if you want a porridge consistency. Less water will give you the consistency of rice.

Simmer and cover with a lid until you have the right consistency, this should roughly take 15–20 minutes or until all the beans, lentils and rice are soft and easily squished.

Serve with salted yoghurt and red onions or poppadom.

LEEK AND POTATO SOUP

  CAN BE MADE VEGETARIAN, VEGAN AND DAIRY FREE

This soup is my mother's love language. Every time I go back to visit her there is a pot of it bubbling away, ready to welcome me, just as there was most weekends when I came home from boarding school as a teenager. It is the soup I make most often for myself to soothe and nourish me in the cold season. We use homemade chicken stock made from a roast chicken carcass from a meal a few days earlier for all the nourishment that this brings, it can of course be made with vegetable stock but will be less hearty in flavour and texture.

Serve with the gluten-free soda bread from earlier in the book or a crusty white loaf. I always have mine with copious amounts of grated cheddar cheese.

Lucy

Serves 4

Two medium leeks, carefully washed, outer leaves and root removed, chopped into 1cm (½in) rounds

One medium onion, finely diced

Three medium potatoes, peeled and cubed

Knob of butter (or oil)

700ml (1½ pints / 3 cups) chicken or vegetable stock

150ml (¼ pint / ¾ cup) of whatever milk you use, or milk and cream mixed

Salt and pepper

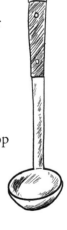

Heat a large saucepan over a medium heat, melt the butter with a tiny splash of oil to stop it burning, add the onions and leeks, stir to cover them in butter and turn the heat down slightly. Cover with a used butter paper or some greaseproof paper and cook for 15–20 minutes until very soft, stirring every few minutes, they shouldn't brown.

Season with salt and pepper, add the potato and stock and cook covered for 20–30 minutes until the potatoes are soft. Add in the milk/cream and check for seasoning.

You can serve it as is, which is my personal preference, or liquidise all or half of it for a thicker, smoother consistency.

Kitchen Witch Magic

Chicken stock or bone broth: sometimes referred to as Jewish penicillin, it has been used for hundreds of years to boost immunity and help nourish convalescents.
Leeks and onions: boost the immune system.
Root vegetables: grounding, they can foster within us a sense of security and safety, supporting any spells of grounding or connection with the root chakra.

COOKING TOGETHER

Often on a Sunday night during the autumn and winter my sister will come over for the afternoon and we will cook together. We cook the sort of dishes that are a hassle to do alone because they are labour intensive. What would be a drag to cook by oneself is so special to prepare together whilst catching up on our news, and such a treat to eat the fruits of our labours: Chinese and Japanese dumplings, Vietnamese spring and summer rolls, steamed Chinese pancakes to go with crispy duck, Indian roti breads to accompany a curry… We sit and chop bowls of vegetables, knead, roll and fill, often joined by some or all of the children. We eat together, play cards or board games, and then wash up together.

During lockdown we also grew a vegetable garden together. Weeding, preparing the ground, planning, planting seeds, watering and harvesting felt like much too onerous a job for either one of us, but together, along with help from my youngest, we created an edible garden to sustain both family households in the uncertainty of the early days of the pandemic.

You may not live close to family, but perhaps there are friends who you can gather with regularly to share cooking, cleaning, eating and play together at each others' houses. When our children were young our group of friends – who had all met via a breastfeeding group – gathered weekly at one house, each bringing a dish to share. We shared achievements and struggles, supported each other, and both parents and children had like-minded company. Now the children are grown we still meet for our seasonal food group, bringing dishes, sharing our lives.

Many communities are starting community kitchens, where people come together and learn new skills, batch cooking healthy meals for their families for the week ahead. Others are creating community gardens where the whole community takes shared responsibility for tending and harvesting an allotment garden.

We wholeheartedly endorse bringing our communities together with and through food, sharing our labour, our wisdom and our support as we nourish each other.

Lucy

Spanish Hot Chocolate

  CAN BE VEGAN, DAIRY FREE

This is the sort of hot chocolate that they make in Spain, thick enough to eat like custard with a spoon, and perfect to dip churros or warm donuts in; any other hot chocolate seems watery to me now!

In my house this is brewed quickly after autumn walks or snowball fights. I serve it as an afterschool treat with freshly made donuts or a weekend brunch with churros. It's also love in a mug if you're pre-menstrual.

Lucy

For each person you will need:

1 teaspoon cocoa + 1 teaspoon sugar (or 40g chocolate – milk to very dark depending on your taste)

¾ teaspoon cornflour (cornstarch)

150ml (5fl oz / ¾ cup) whatever sort of milk you use

Sprinkle of ground cinnamon (optional)

If using cocoa and sugar: Put the milk in a pan and heat through to simmering point. In a cup mix the cornflour, cocoa and sugar together with a couple of tablespoons of cold milk until it forms a smooth paste. Pour half of the hot milk over the top of the paste, stir well, and then tip back into the pan. Bring it to a gentle boil to cook off the cornflour and thicken. Check for sweetness. Pour back into the mug to serve.

If using chocolate: Put the milk and chocolate in a pan and heat through to simmering point. In a cup mix the cornflour with a tablespoon of cold milk until it forms a smooth paste. Pour half of the hot chocolatey milk over the top of the paste, stir well, and then tip back into the pan. Bring it to a gentle boil to cook off the cornflour and thicken. Check for sweetness. Pour back into the mug to serve.

Kitchen Witch Magic: The Cacao Pharmacy

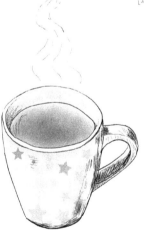

Theobromine: a compound obtained from cacao seeds. It is an alkaloid resembling caffeine in its effects to awaken and enliven.

Magnesium. Some studies have found that taking magnesium supplements could help soothe migraines and PMS symptoms, such as mood swings and bloating (something many women have known intuitively for a long time!)

Tryptophan: found in raw unprocessed cacao, helps our bodies produce serotonin, the neurotransmitter which can support mood, digestion, sleep, memory. You can see how the power of cacao helped it become a ceremonial and healing drink.

Hot Turmeric Milk

  CAN BE VEGAN, DAIRY FREE

I t is probably no surprise to anyone that turmeric is just the best ingredient to have in your home. Ever since I was a child, I have heard my mum utter the words: use turmeric. If I cut myself: put turmeric on it. If I had a cold: have *haldi doodh* (turmeric milk). I have spots: you guessed it, put turmeric on it. This is because turmeric has so many benefits, and the most important one being that it is an anti-inflammatory, which is why it is used in many Indian recipes. Turmeric can help battle colds, aches, pains, helps with healing and overall makes food taste so good.

Even without its benefits, turmeric is regarded highly in Indian households, this is because of its link to Indian mythology. The colour of turmeric is the colour associated with Lord Vishnu, it is believed that the clothes of Lord Vishnu were dyed with turmeric. The yellow-orange colour of the turmeric represents purity and pleasure, combining the colour of the sacral chakra, which represents sensuality and the solar plexus chakra which represents strength and, when aligned, good health.

Khyati Patel

For one healing mug of golden elixir!

Measure out enough full fat milk for your favourite mug (or milk of your choice)

A pinch each of salt, pepper, powdered or freshly grated nutmeg

¼ teaspoon ground turmeric (or grated fresh if you have it)

Honey for sweetening

Bring the milk, turmeric and seasoning to a gentle boil in a pan for a few minutes. Pour into your mug and sweeten with a little honey if desired.

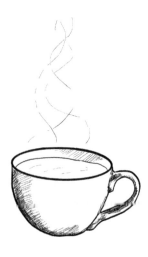

Oatmeal Raisin Cookies

CAN BE GLUTEN-FREE IF USING GLUTEN-FREE OATS AND FLOUR, VEGAN IF REPLACING EGG

These cookies with their comforting oats create delicious smells in the kitchen. Some days are challenging, and when I am feeling the weight of anxiety these cookies help: cinnamon is brave and the raisins are reliable. They pair beautifully with the hot turmeric milk in the previous recipe, for a grown-up kitchen witch version of milk and cookies.

Sarah

Makes 8 cookies

50g (2oz / ⅓ cup) raisins, sultanas or other dried fruit of choice

100g (3½oz / 1 cup) rolled or porridge oats

50g (2oz / ½ cup plain flour) (to make gluten-free, use ½ cup gluten-free or oat flour)

¼ teaspoon bicarbonate of soda

75ml (3fl oz / ⅓ cup) vegetable oil (you can use butter if you prefer)

100g (3½oz / ½ cup) soft brown sugar (caster or granulated sugar work fine too)

1 large egg, beaten (can be swapped for 3 tablespoons maple syrup)

½ teaspoon ground cinnamon

A pinch of salt

Optional for those using an egg: 2 tablespoons honey

Pre-heat the oven to 180°C fan (190°C / 375°F / Gas mark 5).

Mix everything together in a bowl. Roll golf ball sized balls of mixture and then flatten into discs. Pop them on a baking tray lined with baking parchment.

Bake the cookies for about 12–15 minutes or until golden brown around the edges – and the raisins puff up.

Allow to cool a little before enjoying with a hot brew!

Kitchen Witch Magic

Cinnamon: there is a folk myth that says the phoenix builds its nest from cinnamon twigs. Cinnamon in magic can help us make a new start, or to help us pick ourselves up from the ashes.
Raisins: symbolise fertility and the power of the sun, perfect for any kind of creative work.
Oats: to both celebrate and encourage abundance.
Salt: for awareness and protection.

Celebrations

For creative planning with fellow kitchen witches, and any time rain taps on the windows, or the day feels grey…

BRAVE TRUTH COOKIE SPELL

The Chinese have the tradition of fortune cookies: breaking open a cookie after your meal to reveal a line of prophecy. These have been readily taken into Western cultures in Chinese restaurants – we have historically been primed to love divinatory practices, from throwing apple peels to reveal the initial of our future love to hiding charms in celebratory cakes. These cookies are magical in another way.

There exists no precise mix of herbs that will create a tincture to force someone to tell you the truth. You, however, are very much able to create a spell or ritual to help yourself remember your strength, and to support the bravery it takes to ask someone to tell you the truth or to see a truth in a situation. The outcome you seek is not always guaranteed, but you can certainly lay the foundations to success, or to bring you closer to where you wish to be – maybe in this case it is the catalyst to challenging but important conversations…

☾ Fill a bowl with 100g (4oz / 1 cup) of oats.

☾ On top of the bowl place a small dish or candle holder for two candles.

☾ We will use one white candle for truth and one red candle for courage.

☾ Light the candles and passing your hand (safely) over the flames, place your hand to your head and let the heat of your hand linger for a few deep breaths. Then pass it once again over the flames and place your hand to your heart. Finally pass your hand over the flame one last time and bring it to rest on your belly. Then we return to this gesture to the heart, and finally the head. Bringing the energy of truth and bravery to mind, heart and feeling.

☾ Take a final deep breath and gently lift the candles and place them somewhere safe to watch over your work.

☾ Make oatmeal raisin cookies as recipe outlines on previous page (for extra clout from the deities you may want to add the food of the gods: chocolate chunks, or to help words flow, break open a cardamom pod and sprinkle in the tiny seeds).

☽ When your brave truth cookies are ready, lay them out to cool, and blow out your candles.

☽ Use appropriately for your situation. For example:

☆ If you need to have a frank conversation with a friend or colleague, take the cookies with you to eat before, during, or after, or simply as a gift.

☆ If you are heading to a meeting or speaking event and standing in front of a group, eat a cookie with your favourite drink to prepare.

☆ If you are setting off on an adventure, pack a cookie or two to take with you. You may wish to pause on the journey, eat your cookies and ask yourself what you are seeking, or what path is right for you.

☆ Use as an offering at your altar or before a divination practice to explore the truth of a situation or seek a hidden truth.

BLESSING

May love and laughter light your days,
And warm your heart and home.
May good and faithful friends be yours,
Wherever you may roam.
May peace and plenty bless your world
With joy that long endures.
May all life's passing seasons
Bring the best to you and yours!

Traditional Irish Blessing

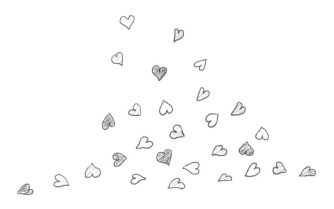

CONCLUSION

Magical cooking and kitchen crafts have a rich and gorgeous history, and, looking forward, reconnecting to them offers us the opportunity to create and consume what we truly hunger for. Whether or not you believe a garden herb or woven poppet can bring prosperity into your life, introducing a little magic into your cooking and time in the kitchen can add meaning and medicine to yourself and all who share your food. There is great joy and comfort to be had in gardening, gathering or shopping for ingredients to bring love, luck, and health to those for whom you cook (and create).

The kitchen is a place that draws elements together – people, ingredients, memories – and through this portal, magic can rise, swell and bubble through the room and through our homes and lives. We all have the capacity to work love and good energy into each meal, and feel nourished by it.

A central concept of kitchen witchery is learning to live consciously and connectedly. We are reminded to cook with the seasons, and honour the cycles of sun and moon in our feasting. To see the potential for magic and enchantment in our daily lives and the places we spend so much of our time. Kitchen witchery reminds us to look again at our lives and the magic behind the mundane, to see food and the kitchen as something special. Whether that's turning food scraps into soup and avoiding food waste, warming an oven pizza to be eaten in front of your favourite film after a challenging day or sharing a candlelit potluck feast with your friends, it can be spiritually fulfilling, delicious and empowering.

The Kitchen Witch reminds us to honour our hunger. And in any act of mindfulness or connection – be it foraging, meditation, stewing or brewing (all of which we have touched on in this journey) – we hope you feel excited to connect to your hunger, to embrace this yearning and dive into new, and old, ways. May you be inspired to seek to satiate all that you hunger for, in the realms of magic in the kitchen.

May you remember always that there is power in your hands: the power to heal, the power to nourish, to tend and grow. You hold within you the gift of transformation as you

cook a recipe and change its ingredients – picking ones that match your mood, season, magical or medicinal needs. You have the power to bless and protect your surroundings, to make the space sacred and
joyful to you and all who enter it. You have the power to create welcome and comfort with what you
have to hand, to foster connection and wellbeing. You can transform what you gather from the wild into
nutritious and tasty goodness.

Thank you for joining us as we have come together in circle, to remember, to learn,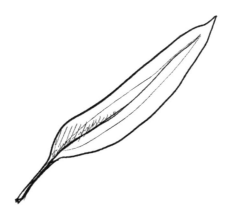
to share our stories, spells and skills. We hope you have found comfort, nourishment
and inspiration from the journey so far. Long may your journey continue. A path of
feeding and fuelling, nourishing and nurturing lies before you. Please seed it with
your own memories, history and culture, what is meaningful and alive for you. Observe the seasonal recipes from your region, savour the seasons as they are where you
live, make notes, forage the wild places and preserve and feast on the goodness you find, grow new
plants, share recipes, seek out ancestral crafts, spells, balms, tinctures, correspondence and wisdom.

Go well, kitchen witch, wise woman, beloved soul, may you always return to your hearth and know
that you are home.

RECIPES

SPELLS AND RITUALS

MEDITATIONS

BIBLIOGRAPHY

Forgotten Skills: The time-honoured ways are the best – over 700 recipes show you why – Darina Allen

The Complete Ballymaloe Cookery Course – Darina Allen

In the Kitchen: essays on food and life – Juliet Annan and Yemisí Aríbisálà

Spirit Weavers: Wisdom Teachings from the Feminine Path of Magic – Seren Bertrand

Culpeper's Complete Herbal – Nicholas Culpeper

The Complete Language of Flowers: A Definitive and Illustrated History – S. Theresa Dietz

Untamed – Glennon Doyle

Plant Lore, Legends, and Lyrics – Richard Folkard

The Herball or Generall Historie of Plantes – John Gerard

River Cafe Cookbook Easy – Rose Gray and Ruth Rogers

Radical Homemakers – Shannon Hayes

The Rise and Fall of Merry England: the ritual year, 1400-1700 – Ronald Hutton

Sacred Celebrations: A Sourcebook – Glennie Kindred

Festivals, Family and Food: A Guide to Seasonal Celebrations – Judy Large and Diana Carey

Witch's Garden: Plants in folklore, magic and traditional medicine – Sandra Lawrence

Healing with Flowers: The Power of Floral Medicine – Anne McIntyre

Jekka's Complete Herb Book – Jekka McVicar

Small Bodies of Water – Nina Mingya Powles

Tiny Moons: A Year of Eating in Shanghai – Nina Mingya Powles

The House Witch: Your Complete Guide to Creating a Magical Space with Rituals and Spells for Hearth and Home – Arin Murphy-Hiscock

The Hedgerow Handbook: Recipes, Remedies and Rituals – Adele Nozedar

Burning Woman – Lucy H. Pearce

Sarah Raven's Complete Christmas Food & Flowers – Sarah Raven

Walking with Persephone: A Journey of Midlife Descent and Renewal – Molly Remer

Kitchen Witch: Food, Folklore & Fairy Tale – Sarah Robinson

Yin Magic: How to be Still – Sarah Robinson

Yoga for Witches – Sarah Robinson

Mystic Cookfire: The Sacred Art of Creating Food to Nurture Friends and Family – Veronika Robinson

The Goddess Celebrates – Diane Stein

A Kitchen Witch's Cookbook – Patricia Talesco

A Spell in the Wild: A Year (and Six Centuries) of Magic – Alice Tarbuck

Dishoom: The first ever cookbook from the much-loved Indian restaurant – Shamil Thakrar and Kavi Thakrar

The Old English Herbals – Eleanour Sinclair Rohde

Witchbody: A Graphic Novel – Sabrina Scott

Magical Food Fiction

The Mistress of Spices – Chitra Divakaruni (Novel)

Like Water for Chocolate – Laura Esquivel (Film) (Novel)

Chocolat – Joanne Harris (Film) (Novel)

Blackberry Wine – Joanne Harris (Novel)

Practical Magic – Alice Hoffman (Film) (Novel)

The Cook of Castamar – Fernando J. Múñez (Netflix Series, based on the novel, *La Cocinera de Castamar*)

Magazines

Enchanted Living, Witch Issue, Autumn 2019

Faerie Magazine, Practical Magic Issue, Autumn 2017

Imaginarium Magazine, August/September 2022

Online

Myth and Moor – Terri Windling

Gather Victoria

Instagram

Brigit Anna McNeill

The Woodland Witchh

Wild Food Love

The Medicine Circle

Must Love Herbs

Jamie Oliver

Facebook

Hedgerow Hermitage

Podcasts

Witch Wednesdays

Missing Witches

Plant Magic

The Magick Kitchen

References from Jacqueline Durban

Cranberry

wikipedia.org/wiki/Cranberry (Vaccinium_macrocarpon) (Vaccinium_oxycoccos)

purecranberry.com/faq/how-do-cranberries-grow

gardeningknowhow.com/edible/fruits/cranberry/do-cranberries-grow-underwater.html

medium.com/think-with-me/cranberry-bog-a946280c2c23

oc.gov/folklife/cranberries/Cranberries.pdf

newenglandfolklore.blogspot.com/2014/7/the-history-of-cranberry-sauce

naturallysimple.org/living/index.php/2019/11/24/cranberryhistory/

researchingfoodhistory.blogspot.com/2013/12/cranberries-on-english-moors-1814.html

shirleytwofeathers.com/the_blog/magickal-ingredients/cranberry-magick-and-lore/

wikipedia.org/wiki/Kalevala

Rowan

wikipedia.org/wiki/Rowan

wikipedia.org/wiki/Sorbus_aucuparia

treesforlife.org.uk/into-the-forest/trees-plants-animals/trees/rowan/

spookyscotland.net/rowan-tree/

somegoodideas.co.uk/articles/the-folklore-and-mythology-of-the-rowan-tree

thehazeltree.co.uk/2013/09/09/the-enchantment-of-the-rowan/

ABOUT THE AUTHORS/ILLUSTRATOR

Sarah Robinson is the best-selling author of *Yoga for Witches* (now available in French, Polish and Chinese), *Yin Magic*, *Kitchen Witch: Food, Folklore & Fairy Tale* which was featured in Cosmopolitan's top witch books and recipient of the Comfy Cosy Book Award 2022, and *Enchanted Journeys*.

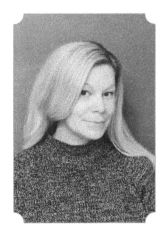

Sarah is a yoga teacher and author based in Bath, UK. Her background is in science, she holds an MSc in Psychology & Neuroscience and has studied at Bath, Exeter and Harvard universities.

Website: sentiayoga.com
Instagram: @yogaforwitches

Lucy H. Pearce is the author of many life-changing non-fiction books, including Nautilus Award winners *Medicine Woman*, *Burning Woman*, and *Creatrix: she who makes*. Her writing focuses on women's healing through archetypal psychology, embodiment, historical awareness and creativity.

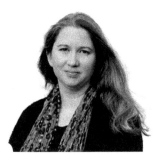

An award-winning graduate in History of Ideas with English Literature from Kingston University, and a PGCE from Cambridge University, Lucy founded Womancraft Publishing, publishing paradigm-shifting books by women for women, in 2014. The mother of three children, she lives in a small village by the Celtic Sea in East Cork, Ireland.

Lucy is a multi-faceted creative whose work spans the expressive arts, exploring the lost archetypes of the feminine and symbols of the soul. As a long time enthusiast of all things herbal and hedgerow, she truly enjoyed the process of creating the internal illustrations for this book.

Website: lucyhpearce.com / womancraftpublishing.com
Instagram: @lucyhpearce

ABOUT THE COVER ARTIST

Jessica Roux is a Nashville-based freelance illustrator and plant and animal enthusiast. She loves exploring in her own backyard and being surrounded by an abundance of nature. Using subdued colours and rhythmic shapes, she renders flora and fauna with intricate detail reminiscent of old world beauty.

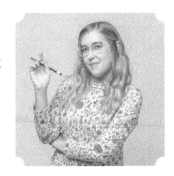

Website: jessica-roux.com Instagram: @jessicasroux

ABOUT WOMANCRAFT

Womancraft Publishing was founded on the revolutionary vision that women and words can change the world. We act as midwife to transformational women's words that have the power to challenge, inspire, heal and speak to the silenced aspects of ourselves, empowering our readers to actively co-create cultures that value and support the female and feminine. Our books have been #1 Amazon bestsellers in many categories, as well as Nautilus and Women's Spirituality Award winners.

As we find ourselves in a time where old stories, old answers and ways of being are losing their authority and relevance, we at Womancraft are actively looking for new ways forward. Our books ask important questions. We aim to share a diverse range of voices, of different ages, backgrounds, sexual orientations and neurotypes, seeking every greater diversity, whilst acknowledging our limitations as a small press.

At the heart of our Womancraft philosophy is fairness and integrity. Creatives and women have always been underpaid: not on our watch! We split royalties 50:50 with our authors. We offer support and mentoring throughout the publishing process as standard. We use almost exclusively female artists on our covers, and as well as paying fairly for these cover images, offer a royalty share and promote the artists both in the books and online. Whilst far from perfect, we are proud that in our small way, Womancraft is walking its talk, living the new paradigm in the crumbling heart of the old: through financially empowering creative people, through words that honour the Feminine, through healthy working practices, and through integrating business with our lives, and rooting our economic decisions in what supports and sustains our natural environment. We are learning and improving all the time. I hope that one day soon, what we do is seen as nothing remarkable, just the norm.

We work on a full circle model of giving and receiving: reaching backwards, supporting Treesisters' reforestation projects and the UNHCR girls' education fund, and forwards via Worldreader, providing e-books at no-cost to education projects for girls and women in developing countries. We donate many paperback copies to education projects and women's libraries around the world. We speak from our place within the circle of women, sharing our vision, and encouraging them to share it onwards, in ever-widening circles.

We are honoured that the Womancraft community is growing internationally year on year, seeding red tents, book groups, women's circles, ceremonies and classes into the fabric of our world. Join the revolution! Sign up to the mailing list at womancraftpublishing.com and find us on social media for exclusive offers:

 womancraftpublishing

 womancraftbooks

 womancraft_publishing

**Signed copies of all titles available from
shop.womancraftpublishing.com**

USE OF WOMANCRAFT WORK

Often women contact us asking if and how they may use our work. We love seeing our work out in the world. We love you sharing our words further. And we ask that you respect our hard work by acknowledging the source of the words.

We are delighted for short quotes from our books – up to 200 words – to be shared as memes or in your own articles or books, provided they are clearly accompanied by the author's name and the book's title.

We are also very happy for the materials in our books to be shared amongst women's communities: to be studied by book groups, discussed in classes, read from in ceremony, quoted on social media… with the following provisos:

☾ If content from the book is shared in written or spoken form, the book's author and title must be referenced clearly.

☾ The only person fully qualified to teach the material from any of our titles is the author of the book itself. There are no accredited teachers of this work. Please do not make claims of this sort.

☾ If you are creating a course devoted to the content of one of our books, its title and author must be clearly acknowledged on all promotional material (posters, websites, social media posts).

☾ The book's cover may be used in promotional materials or social media posts. The cover art is copyright of the artist and has been licensed exclusively for this book. Any element of the book's cover or font may not be used in branding your own marketing materials when teaching the content of the book, or content very similar to the original book.

☾ No more than two double page spreads, or four single pages of any book may be photocopied as teaching materials.

We are delighted to offer a 20% discount of over five copies going to one address. You can order these on our webshop, or email us. If you require further clarification, email us at: info@womancraft-publishing.com